TAKE THAT NURSING HOME AND SHOVE IT!

Cenlyt Dennis I miss you and only hope that you are well Love Seven

(310)
897-
7434

TAKE THAT NURSING HOME AND SHOVE IT!

How to Secure
an Independent
Future for Yourself
and Your Loved Ones

SUSAN B. GEFFEN

Gerontologist, Elder Law Attorney

Take That Nursing Home and Shove It!

Published by Sage Press
Redondo Beach, CA

ISBN: 978-0-9842160-1-7

For more information about the author or to contact her:
www.susanbgeffen.com
310-406-0608

Printed in the United States of America

ACKNOWLEDGMENTS

I would like to acknowledge my husband Joel Geffen. He is my best friend, husband and the only person who has ever believed in me and pushed me to reach my potential. He along with my kids have had to put up with the stress involved in writing a 300-plus page book and for them I have the deepest love in my heart.

I would also like to acknowledge author Tom Sullivan, who graciously mentored me through the beginning phases of this process and who told me that in order to connect with the readers I had to reveal some of my own personal challenges.

Of course, my friend JC, who is like the mother I never had, gets a big thanks for supporting me through the process of writing this book, as does my friend and colleague Florie Leddel, long-term care insurance expert, who guided me on that important piece of the book. My client Steve, deserves a nod for meticulously looking at my punctuation and grammar. I would also like to thank Linda Weber, the librarian at USC, for forgiving me for the loss of 12 books I checked out and were inadvertently tossed into the trash before I had a chance to return them.

I also thank the universe for blessing me with the good mind and health to be able to persevere.

Table of Contents

"It is not the strongest of the species that survive, nor the most intelligent, but the one most responsive to change."
—Charles Darwin

INTRODUCTION

I am an elder law attorney and gerontologist. Many ask why I chose to write a book that picks on the nursing home industry. Many have suggested that I am committing career suicide by choosing to go down this path because the nursing home lobby is very large and powerful. I am leaving myself vulnerable to attacks from many stakeholders. Yet, for me it was a no brainer. Why? Because a significant portion of us soon-to-be-older adults will end up in nursing homes if we don't start to formulate our plans. *They are not the best place for you or me.* This book will help you stay out of a nursing home or choose the right one, should that be your only option.

I want people to understand that the term "nursing home" is an oxymoron. Nursing homes smell bad. Does your home smell like sick people and Fabuloso, the dollar store disinfectant? Nursing homes look like a hybrid of high school and the hospital. I could not wait to escape from the former as it was terribly boring and oppressed my freedom to engage in the most basic of rights (such as going to the bathroom without first raising my hand); I never want to be in the latter.

Almost 2 million older Americans live in nursing homes. Most of these places (if not all) are understaffed, and statistics consistently demonstrate that older adults are abused and neglected in them. Almost 25 percent of the nation's nursing facilities deliver poor care and cause harm and jeopardy to their residents. This "harm" includes death. When I get a call from an adult son who tells me that a facility lost his father's teeth and then continued to feed him solid food on which he choked and aspirated, I *want* to crucify the industry. I get these types of calls all of the time. In my opinion, nursing homes are like a lobster's house at Delmonico's—a holding tank before death.

This book is not really about indicting the nursing home industry, although I clearly believe it is highly indictable. Rather, it is meant to help you age on your own terms. For most people that means with dignity and independence, but life in a nursing home allows neither. I am going to ask that you put your trust in me for the remainder of this book. I can personally guarantee that when you are finished reading it, you will no longer think of a nursing home as a potential housing option or fear that you will spend the remaining days of your life in one. You can count on me and all that I have written to clear the path to financial and personal independence.

Now for the harsh criticism that supports the title of this book: Most nursing homes are disgusting. They live up to the image they conjure. There is no time to speak with a delicate voice; I must be unapologetically blunt. If I could reach my hand out from this book and slap reality into four generations of sleepwalkers, I would. If I could afford to take out billboards across

Route 66 warning people that the danger of complacency is being relegated to a foul smelling nightmare in their old age, I would. But I can't do either of these, because one is just an imaginary impulse and the other is too costly. However, I can write.

I was once told by a literary agent that my writing sounds angry, but she could not understand the difference between passion and anger. I am passionate because of my compassion. I would not and will not be stifled, and that is why I refused to change the title or tone of my book. I can effectuate massive change by publishing a book that gives people a road map of how to steer clear of nursing homes and how to stay healthy. After all, what is the point of "100 is the new 70" if our minds are mush, our bodies frail, our finances depleted, and our surroundings bleak?

You do not have to end up in one of these facilities if you have a plan. This book will challenge you to get off your duff and develop your own exit plan, or at a minimum, acknowledge that at some point the jig will be up and it's the journey that counts. A little spiritual psychobabble never hurt anyone. This book will give you as many tools as I can personally provide to ensure that your future—our collective future—is *lovely*. That is a good word, *lovely*. As weary travelers on this planet, that is what we deserve: a lovely elder life journey and conclusion. Again, please trust me when I say that by the end of this book, you will be able to figure out how to stay out of a nursing home and afford to live the life you deserve.

Like many Americans, I have worked hard. I put myself through college, law school, and graduate school. I have overcome obstacles and I know that life is like a fragile necklace, bound together by alternating beads of sorrow and utter joy. I am middle aged, well-educated, healthy, I live in a nice middle-class neighborhood and yet, I am frightened by what I see. I see my future unfolding every day as I meet with old, frail human beings in one stage of chronic illness or another. For the unlucky, this can be a long arduous journey, like a Friday rush hour on the 405 freeway. We don't want to think or speak of it. However, unless we are blessed with a quick ending, *it can be very humiliating*. What upsets me more is that **it does not have to be that way for anyone**.

Too often, we live by a "that is not going to happen to me" mentality and therefore do not plan. Like me, most of the older adults I meet lived rich, full lives, and this is at the heart of my own fear. No matter what they look like or what their gender, I see myself in them. The reflection in their mirror always looks like me, albeit an older version. I want to help them because *I am them*. We share fate, and all that is different between us is a nebulous concept of time. Each of us knows that those are not hands we can turn back.

Many people ask me why I have this extreme empathic nature. I was treated unjustly as a child. I was physically attacked by my brother, who is four years my senior. How a little sister could provoke a tall, strong boy into hitting her and throwing her and twisting her like a licorice Twizzler has always escaped me. I was wrongfully accused and verbally abused by my mother and I grew up hearing that I was a mistake that my mother should have aborted. Until her death three years ago, I was still "nothing but a disappointment." My father, with whom I am very close, was no prize either. He *was* a philanderer, gambler and cheat. (Sorry dad, but this is for education.) My parents' divorce when I was 12 was a welcome relief from the screaming and violence that forced me into my big sister's bed every night. Lest you glean that I am still hurt, I am not. I find tremendous value in going to a place of love in my heart for all those who have bruised my innards. Doing so feels like going on a vacation, although the sojourn can be like taking a grueling flight with many layovers!

One summer in my childhood, I had the luxury of agonizing for hours on end over the fate of a fly who buzzed around my mother's car from my home in the suburbs to my grandmother's home in the city. Concerned with its ability to adjust to a new environment and new friends, I barraged my mother with questions designed to secure information regarding the fly's future. Because I feared that the fly would have no way to communicate its whereabouts to its family, I refused to open the car's windows. It would just have to sit and wait in the car during the drive and until our visit was over and we could bring it back to my neighborhood, its neighborhood.

The heat was stifling and my mother's 1973 gold Plymouth Duster was fogged in with smoke emanating from her filterless Pall Malls. Nevertheless, I persevered. *What if it can't find its way home?* In retrospect, the fact that I chose heat prostration and smoke inhalation for the sake of a tiny bug indicates to me that my heart has bled since childhood for those without a voice. I believe that being perceived like an undeserving little person myself contributed to this fight in me. I want to help people; I always have and I always will. It is an inexplicable reaction I have to injustice. I feel others' pain as if it were driven into my own guts.

Indeed, I have always stood up for the underdog—my buck-toothed neighbor, the scrawny schlep, the cherubic child. I specifically recall carrying on with summer rituals such as kick the can, running bases, and statue maker, all the while defending these underdogs. If someone was getting picked on, I inevitably felt the urge to intercede. It did not matter if the bully was older than me, or if he was a boy. Whoever was picking on the defenseless nerd would have to put up their dukes. I had learned how to fight well from fending off the brutal attacks by my older brother and basically, by age ten, I could beat up anybody within a two-year range—or at least I thought so.

For a good portion of my career as an attorney, I tried to help the disabled and aged by litigating discrimination cases. Now that I have a master's of science degree in gerontology, I am able to assist families with both the legal and social aspects of aging. I am driven to help the baby boomers and beyond through individual consultations, educational lectures and, now, by writing this book. This is not a step-by-step guide on how to thwart death. It is a book that will give you every single item that you need to know about aging successfully. Like everything else that I do, I have poured my heart and soul into this piece. I do so with love, for all of you.

You may have heard that the percentage of elderly living in nursing homes is on the decline. This is true, but it is because people are experiencing better health and because there is a proliferation of more attractive housing for those who are financially able to afford the fees they charge. However, we are on the precipice of an "age tsunami": by 2050, 90 million Americans will be over 65. This is unprecedented and therefore we cannot just ignore these aging statistics with their concomitant chronic conditions, like I ignore the unpaid parking tickets scattered around my home. Unless this cohort of Americans, myself among them, engages in a dialogue about what to expect out of the later years, and demands the right to be treated with dignity in the least restrictive environment, I do not expect nursing home occupancy to continue to decline. Instead, we will need more places to house the frail older adults of the future. If we live long enough, we will become frail.

I will also gladly admit that there are *some* reputable nursing homes all across the country. There are a lot of honest proprietors trying to do a good job despite many obstacles. In the pursuit of fairness and balance, I will explore how to find these facilities. Nonetheless, by and large, they are not where anyone wants to be. So, I hereby publicly vow never to *live* in a nursing home. (I can say that because I have formulated a plan. By the end of this book, you will have too.)

There exist recent data and studies that show that regulatory mechanisms do not do enough to combat the problems of nursing home abuse and neglect. A recent government study found that 30 percent of nursing homes in the United States—5,283 facilities—were cited for almost 9,000 instances of abuse between January 1999 and January 2001. These problems include untreated bedsores, inadequate medical care, malnutrition, dehydration, preventable accidents, and substandard sanitation and hygiene. According to that report, in 1,601 of these cases the nursing home abuse violations were serious enough "to cause actual harm to residents or to place the residents in immediate jeopardy of death or serious injury."[1]

Not much has changed since then. In 2009, approximately 156,000 deficiencies were issued to nursing homes for violations of federal regulations; 24.7 percent of the nation's nursing facilities received deficiencies for poor quality of care, where they caused harm or jeopardy to residents. This was a 3 percent increase over 2004, which shows that poor quality of care continues to be a major problem in the United States.[2] According to a 2011 University of California, San Francisco study of the 10 largest national for-profit chains, it is primarily the *for-profit* industry that does not adequately staff its homes and that delivers the lowest quality of care.[3]

Let me say it again: **You do not have to end up in a nursing home if you have a plan, a voice, and the impetus to use it**. Let's appreciate nursing homes for what they do best— rehabilitate people and then get them the hell out.

This is not meant to be a high brow academic exposition. It is an impassioned plea by an educated, caring person. In my role as a family elder care consultant,[4] I see family after family struggling with what to do about a spouse or an ailing parent. I am almost always called when things are in a crisis mode. Typically, a parent or spouse is getting discharged from a hospital stay and there is no plan, only sheer panic. If there were no solution to this recurring dilemma, I would pack up my laptop and go play poker, which is what I do when I want to avoid responsibility. But, there are steps that we can take to mitigate this pain and confusion.

In some places I will ask you to concentrate on regulations that, as a consumer, you need to understand. I equivocated about discussing some of the convoluted governmental systems at play, but then concluded that it just may be my purpose to deconstruct them so that they do not remain inaccessible. All of us need to know how Medicare and Medicaid reimburse and regulate nursing homes. Otherwise, how can we move the government toward responsible action?

This book also explores alternatives to nursing homes, including the technologies that will enable us to stay in our own homes longer and that help families engage in long-distance caregiving. I also describe innovative programs being developed at the grass roots level that can provide templates for every community to care for their elderly constituents. I will discuss laws that allow people to leave work to care for loved ones, such as the Family Medical Leave Act (FMLA), and laws that prohibit age discrimination in the workplace, such as the Age Discrimination in Employment Act (ADEA).

According to a 2011 study by the SCAN Foundation and the UCLA Center for Health Policy Research, 66 percent of voters aged 40 and older cannot afford more than three months of nursing home care. After reading this book, you will not be able to claim that you did not know that care was so expensive, or that you are statistically likely to need these services after reaching the age of 65. Every way to finance this care will be revealed.

This book also offers empirical data to prove that good physical and mental health habits can thwart the development of most chronic diseases, including Alzheimer's disease. Those habits are delineated.

My objective is to motivate you to take responsibility for your personal and our collective futures, to cajole you into becoming more educated and politically active so as to influence public policy. If you follow my lead, we old folks of the future will be exactly what we want to be: Pacman-playing, concert-going, traveling, healthy, fit fools.

CHAPTER 1

Wake Up and Smell the Reality

Merriam-Webster tells us that a pandemic is something that occurs over a wide geographic area and affects an exceptionally high proportion of the population. There is currently a pandemic of ignorance in America. Few know that 70 percent of people over age 65 will require at least some long-term care services during their lifetime and others mistakenly believe they will be covered by resources that actually do not pay for such care.[5] This is meaningful information, yet the average American is totally unaware. We need to wake up and smell the reality.

The cost of long-term care is significant. The *MetLife Long-Term Care IQ Survey*, completed by 1,021 individuals aged 40 to 70, reveals that most of us are not taking appropriate steps to protect ourselves from potentially catastrophic expenses. If you do not have money or insurance, what will you do when these statistics beckon you? When they knock on your door, you will be knocking on the nursing home door, because that is where poor people go when they need care.

Please do not put this book down while you utter under your breath, "I am not poor." I assure you that such words rolled off the tongues of millions of people in this country who now wonder if they will outlive their money. Those who are educated and worked their whole lives, those who traveled to countless destinations and stayed in four-star resorts are now facing futures in dumps. Are you feeling uncomfortable or scared yet? Good. I want you to feel something so that you will keep reading and then take action to prepare yourself for living life on your own terms!

I have seven *very* sophisticated theories about why we ignore the truth about our future:

Hypothesis 1: Brain Freeze

Our society suffers from analysis paralysis. We are constantly exposed to overwhelming volumes of information, and information fatigue syndrome hampers our decision-making abilities. There is an abundance of information available to us on almost every subject, including aging. This information increases at such a rapid pace that tracking, understanding, and integrating it requires a great deal of time and effort. At the same time, we have expectations of having instant access to information that, in sound bite fashion, gives us just what we think we need to understand any given subject. We are taken to the precipice of knowledge and seek no further elucidation. Information from research is not automatically converted into meaningful knowledge, and knowledge is not automatically transferred into practice.

This paradox has been referred to as the "knowing–doing gap,"[6] and the result is disorientation and a lack of responsiveness. In 1965, when a host of technological and social changes were occurring in the United States, Alvin Toffler posited information overload as having the same sort of effects, but on higher cognitive functions: "When the individual is plunged into a fast and irregularly changing situation, or a novelty-loaded context…his predictive accuracy plummets. He can no longer make the reasonably correct assessments on which rational behavior is dependent."[7]

In this information age, it is easy to shut down. Unfortunately, you cannot afford to bury yourself under that onslaught. You *have to* dive in head first and cull through legal, financial, medical, and public policy issues. If you don't, your chances of being institutionalized when you are older are much greater. By reading on, you will be one step closer to understanding exactly what you need to do to ensure that you are on the right path to successful aging.

Hypothesis 2: We Are the Bologna

It is easy to lose yourself and the focus of your future in the frenzy of attending to daily tasks, especially if you are part of the sandwich generation. Nearly 10 million baby boomers are now raising kids or supporting adult children while also giving a financial hand to aging parents, the Pew Research Center reports. Seventy percent of this generation is simultaneously taking care of their parents and children, both of whom are vying for physical and financial attention. If that is you, you are the bologna.

A University of Southern California Leonard Davis School of Gerontology study concluded that baby boomers "are even more committed to caring for aging parents than their own parents were." And while women are typically seen as the primary caregivers in this group, in my practice I hear from equal numbers of men and women who are struggling as they navigate this complex relationship. Members of the sandwich generation are responsible for intra-family wealth transfers on the order of $18 billion and 2.4 billion hours each year.[8] Building on the metaphor, professionals now refer to the generation that cares for their children, grandchildren, and parents as the club sandwich generation. If you are in this position it is almost impossible to get a light snack at a mini market, let alone make a living. Even more difficult is getting other people to understand what you are going through. If you are one of these caregivers, how are you supposed to think about anything other than what is on your plate? How are you supposed to focus on your future and financial stability when your daily routine consists of putting out fires and avoiding one emergent situation after another? You are like Dorothy, swirling around in the eye of the tornado.

Dorothy could not figure out how to get home until she was knocked unconscious in a poppy field. Here is something that should awaken you from your busy bee spell: In present dollars, bills for a stay in a nursing home or assisted-living facility or for extended home care can easily reach $50,000 to $100,000 a year or more. I am no economist but I think it will only get more expensive. As much as you want to support your parents, it is imperative that you put saving for your retirement first. Have I mentioned that you do not want to end up in a nursing home?

Hypothesis 3: I Am Going to Die Soon Anyway

Guess what? You are not going to die soon. In 1950, when those in the first wave of boomers were mere babes, only 56 percent of men and 65 percent of women were expected to live past the age of 65. But the fastest-growing segment of the total population is the oldest—those 80 and over. The growth rate of this population segment is twice that of those 65 and over and almost four times that of the total population. In the United States, this group now represents 10 percent of the older population and will *more than triple* from 5.7 million in 2010 to over 19 million by 2050.

When I was growing up I recall people talking about saving for their retirement, a utopian paradise marked by cruises to exotic destinations and golf in Scotland; an idyllic world in which to live out one's golden years. Now, one of the saddest things for me to manage is answering the all-too-often asked question, "Am I going to outlive my money?" This question comes from older adults who have worked hard their entire lives, enjoyed the afore-mentioned perks of saving for retirement, and who are now in their nineties. They are in need of assistance in the home or they need to move to another, more suitable location. Perhaps they can no longer live in their homes because they cannot afford the rent or they have already used the equity in their homes to finance the last 10 years of their lives. Some have spent it on a spouse whose health declined and now they must go without. Many of these people will find themselves in Medicaid beds in nursing home facil-ities if their children do not take them in.

I was called to a 94-year-old woman's apartment in Marina Del Rey. Her son called me because she had $27,000 left on which to live. Her rent was $2,000 a month and her live-in caregiver $6,000 a month. Her son was managing her money and I am convinced that at all times he was trying to honor his mother's wishes. She had COPD and congestive heart failure. She was frail but very much with it. I held her hand and after I explained that she needed to give notice of intent to move, she said, "I really did not think that I was going to live this long." Now, both of her children will need to supplement her limited Social Security and I will guide them with benefits. If she had a plan, she would have been comfort-able for the rest of her life. As it stands, I helped them find a comfortable place, but the move will be very difficult for her.

Another couple, both in their early seventies, called me. The husband's Parkinson's disease, which he had lived with for 15 years, *had been progressing slowly, but now he needed $1,500 a month for in-home care. They also paid $2,000 each month in rent. After my calculations, it turned out that if everything stayed the same, they would have 13 years of money left. However, she had a part-time job that she could no longer sustain, and his level and cost of care would most assuredly increase. Even if there was a modest 50 percent increase in their living expenses, they would have only seven years of money left. As I left she fretted, "I have longevity on my side, my mother is in her nineties and my father passed away in his late eighties."*

While I am not preaching pleasure deferral, and spiritually there is much to be said for living in the present, sometimes we have to peek our heads out and glance at the future. This is that time. I just ask that you check in on it once in a while as if it were a sleeping tiger whose surprise awakening could mean the difference between a lovely spectacle of grace and an unfortunate calamity.

Hypothesis 4: We Are Hard Wired to Avoid Pain

Many of the choices we make in our daily lives are motivated by the potential for two powerful forces—pleasure and pain. We are obviously attracted to that which causes pleasure and we avoid what causes pain. I think it is safe to say that there are many aspects of our years as octogenarians that we do not associate with pleasure. Otherwise, people would not choose to get face lifts or buy anti-aging products—parts of an industry predicted to generate profits of nearly $292 billion by 2015. In fact, we not only avoid the truth when it is painful—at times, it is human nature to *deny* it. Again, that is a choice. Instead of embracing our age, many people hold onto their youth like mountain climbers to their rope. If they let go, they spiral into the abyss of old age and suffer the consequences that it inevitably brings. But this is a very destructive way to proceed, spurred by an uninformed thought process.

I AM ALMOST 50. THERE, I SAID IT. I HAVE WRINKLES AND STRETCH MARKS AND CELLULITE AND GRAY ROOTS THAT I DYE EVERY SIX WEEKS. I HAVE HAIR GROWING ON PLACES ON MY FACE THAT MAKE ME QUESTION IF I EVER PRODUCED ESTROGEN. *THAT FELT SO GOOD!*

Putting a pillow over your head does not change what is inevitable. Being honest with yourself, and then taking action, does.

Hypothesis 5: That Is Not Me, That Is Someone Else

"Suze, your old man ain't going anywhere," said my dad. He is 82. My response, "Really, how did you arrange that? Is there someone who I need to talk to? Is it a genetic thing?" He had no estate plan. He had no plan. He is Bert the Great.

Guess what? It happened to him. And, because he had no plan, it happened to me. When it happened, I flushed the catheter that was attached to his penis every four hours, emptied urine from another two bags, changed his sheets and pajamas three times a day, cleaned the carpet from him because he leaked. My husband bathed him and often cleaned the feces off of the floor (that I stepped in as I followed him to the bathroom so he would not fall) because he had to take an enema and was too weak to make it to the bathroom in a timely manner. But for the fact that my father was rehabilitating from having his bladder and prostate removed and there was an end in sight, I do not think that it was a sustainable situation. Sorry dad, but—like I said—this is for education.

Hypothesis 6: We Are Zombies

I believe that far too often we walk around in a somnambulistic state uttering the mantra, "The government will take care of us." If you think that the folks in Washington, D.C., will sprinkle fairy dust onto the playing field and magically transform our futures into a financially secure, medically stable, housing friendly utopia then maybe you should return this book and get your money back. The characters in twenty-first century zombie flicks may be cool to look at, but being bereft of consciousness and self-awareness about the government's constraints is downright dangerous.

It is imperative that you understand the impact of the coming accelerated swell of older adults because it will have a significant impact on the cost of providing health services.[9] Ask yourself this: If Medicare, the trust fund for the health insurance system for the elderly, runs out of money in the next ten years as is slated, how are our medical and hospital bills going to get paid? This is not insignificant. Starting in 2011, 10,000 people in the United States will turn 65 years old every day. There will be another ten years of people turning 65 at comparable rates after that. For almost 50 decades, Americans have looked forward to availing themselves of Medicare benefits like a trapeze acrobat to the forthcoming swing, but it is no longer that simple. Our level of health care now correlates directly to our age.

If you just take from this book that there is a difference between Medicare and Medicaid, you are one step closer to staying out of a nursing home. You will read that Medicare does not pay for long-term care and that Medicaid will pay for your food and housing and care in a nursing home (yuck), but you will have to be dirt poor to get this assistance. If you are not yet clear on the differences between these two social programs, you are not alone; most individuals with whom I speak do not know the differences between them either. Can you imagine finding out at the eleventh hour that you grossly misunderstood the role of Medicare in your fantasy of the government's role in protecting you? It is essential that you do not continue on in a zombie-like state, without the information that can help you chart your path.

Hypothesis 7: It Is None of Your Damned Business

Whether by design or by circumstance, many of us will approach our golden years with our adult children as our partners. The more we can engage them in this process from the earliest stages, the more helpful they can be. Unfortunately, the number one question I hear from adult children of aging parents: How can I get my parents to talk to me about these important issues? The number one tragedy I see? Adult children in the throes of rapid-fire decision making while trying to adapt to a parent's sudden onset of Alzheimer's or dementia. I get calls from adult children whose parents are getting discharged from a hospital or rehabilitation facility and they have no idea what to do next. They are crying. Yes, your adult children are crying. They are mostly your daughters, but the wonderful sons that I meet hold in their tears, clinging to their own bodies when we speak. Many feel shame at their helplessness. They want to fix the problem and it is too late. They will carry this guilt with them forever.

Because of your adult children's caregiving responsibilities, they will get to work late, have to leave early, have phone interruptions from medical personnel or confused parents, and perhaps get fired or demoted. This would be tragic. A study that was done several years ago found a sizeable number of families went into bankruptcy over caring for their families. This would be tragic. Worse, they can become so tired that they are at higher risk for illness or accidents. They could die.[10] This would be tragic. Clearly I am not mincing words here; political correctness will not get you to do the following, in this order:

1. Grant power of attorney for your finances.

Power of attorney authorizes another individual to act for you in legal, financial, or health care matters if you are unable to do so. If you have not already granted power of attorney to another trusted individual for your finances, do so immediately, and then tell your children where your money is and who the agent is. This can save you from being the subject of a conservatorship/guardianship (in some states they are called different things), which is a costly endeavor and could pit family members against one another and can keep you from getting the care that you need.

I met with a woman and her brother about her parents. The mother's Alzheimer's disease was progressing rapidly. The father was frail. Their parents refused to discuss the details of their finances with them. The parents had a house that had a reverse mortgage and that was all they knew. There was no estate plan in place, no trust, no will. There was an advance health care directive, and the daughter was a co-agent with her brother. No one except the spouses had access to the funds.

Within three months, the father was in the hospital on a ventilator and the neighbors were on the verge of calling adult protective services because the mother called the neighbors at all hours of the night screaming, "my husband is dead." Then, she began to wander. There were two choices. The police could come and get the mother and she would be put in a psychiatric ward and then circulated back and forth through a broken system, or the daughter could have her placed into an Alzheimer's facility. Since the father was unconscious, and the mother was unable to contribute to a conversation about how to pay for her care, the daughter began to pay $6,000 a month out of her own pocket until the financial matters got resolved. The woman's father died shortly thereafter. The daughter had to move for a conservatorship.

The mother wanted to get out of the facility. She fought the conservatorship and she and her daughter became adversaries. This cost the estate thousands and thousands of dollars. The court required three doctors to certify that this woman's mother was too cognitively disabled to manage her affairs and countless in-court proceedings ensued. Because she had some fleeting moments of lucidity, the court had to be very prudent in carefully balancing this woman's right to independence and autonomy against the possibility that she would be neglected if left to her own devices. This kind daughter is broke and broken now.

Sometimes, all of the parent's money or assets are in a trust. If this is the case, a simple power of attorney for finances might not help. Let's assume, for example, that a father is the grantor (creator) and trustee of his trust, the individual who can manage the property or assets within it. Now, let's assume that the father has dementia and there is no successor trustee identified. Nobody will be able to reach the assets to pay for his care without court intervention. In this case, only a successor trustee would be able to act on the incapacity of the grantor. If you have a trust, make sure that you name successor trustees who can access your property in case you become too disabled to do so yourself.

Many clients confide that they are joint tenants on their parents' checking accounts and/or property. Parents: this may not be such a good idea. Aside from the potential unintended gift taxes (although at this time there is a $5 million lifetime exemption), suppose you own a bank account with your child to make it easy for him to write out the checks for your bills. This enables your child to write out a check for everything that is in the account and pay off his debts. You will not be able to stop him from doing so, as he is legally an owner of that account, even though he didn't contribute a penny to it.

But for an unexpected inheritance, one of my clients would have been rendered destitute by her son who took a reverse mortgage out on her house and kept the proceeds. When I called him to find out where the money had gone, he stated that he used it to pay his bills. I guess he either did not care that I was an elder law attorney or did not comprehend the nature of his financial abuse. However, by the time the conversation was over, I believed that he got the message. It would not take much to do so as I bluntly told him, "you committed elder abuse against your 95-year-old mother." Because he had used all of the money for his own benefit (as is usually the case), I could not get it back for her. She loved her son and, even though she knew that he almost destroyed her, she would not press charges. Almost six months later, after I had her put a new agent in charge of her finances, her son called her and suggested that she open a joint checking account with him. When I called him, I suggested that he learn how to cope with life in a small cell with a public urinal.

I wish I could tell you that these are isolated incidents—that you can simply trust your child or loved one to act in your own best interests. But these things happen more often than you or I would like to admit, and you need to know that as you plan for your financial future.

Last year I was asked to draft a woman's will by her adult daughter. Of course, I could not do so unless I met with her mother alone and was retained by her mother. However, it turned out that a will was unnecessary. The mother had placed her daughter on her $700,000 checking account as a joint tenant. In this case, the joint tenancy meant that both she and her daughter had an equal right to the $700,000 during each other's lives. At the death of the mother, the money would belong to the daughter without any court intervention.

The mother, a Holocaust survivor, did not have the capacity to change her will anyway. The daughter, who was in charge of her care, placed her mother in a shared room at a facility that made me vomit when I left. She wanted to preserve the money in the account for her own use. She saved $5,000 a month by placing her mother in a dirty home. All I could do was to rip up the daughter's retainer check and tell her that she was the scum of the earth.

Placing your children's names on the deed to your home as a joint tenant might make it easier for them to inherit your house, but it could hinder your ability to *sell* the property, should you need or wish to do so. If you desire to sell your home and use the funds to pay for assisted living, your children will have to sign the deed. Without their signatures (because they are owners too), you cannot sell. You cannot get a home equity loan or reverse mortgage without their signatures on the loan documents. They have the right to live in the house even if you don't want them living there. And, in a community property state, if one of your children's spouses is divorcing your child, that spouse can have a claim against your house (because the spouse that he/she is divorcing is one of the owners). Additionally, the person assuming "the gift" of joint ownership will lose the step-up in basis at death (the income tax valuation of inherited assets at the time of death vs. time of purchase) and capital gains taxes may have to be paid. If the property is not the principal residence of the new tenant, the capital gains exclusion will not be available either.

As with your checking account, if your child loses a lawsuit and has a judgment filed against him, your home will be subject to the judgment creditor. Now that creditor can own your property in satisfaction of the judgment against your child. Also, there is the possibility that your child could become mentally or physically disabled and unable to sign documents. If the incapacitated child has not appointed an attorney-in-fact using a durable power of attorney, you cannot sell, mortgage, or gift your property until you go to court to get a conservator appointed for the other joint owner. As you know now, this is expensive and time consuming.

If I had a dollar for every time I was told by a spouse or adult child that they just transferred money out of their spouse's or parent's account to allow them to "qualify" for Medicaid, I would have enough money to take my family to Denny's for dinner. (What can I say? A dollar does not buy much lately.) I will delve into this subject in a later chapter, but suffice it to say that, in most states, you must redo a title or transfer assets at least five years prior to a Medicaid claim in order to avoid what are called "look back" rules and sanctions on any gift to a non-spouse owner. Money transferred into a joint account is not considered a valid transfer for Medicaid either. Unless you can demonstrate that the joint tenant placed his or her own money into the account, the entire balance will be counted for eligibility purposes. The point is that this type of "planning" may impact the receipt of public benefits. If your actions do not satisfy these "look back" rules, benefits could be *delayed for years*. Even worse—and more relevant to the subject at hand—if the transferee absconds with the funds, you will have no money for your care and no sympathy from the eligibility worker. Even if there is no malfeasance (though there often is), the eligibility worker could accuse the transferee and the attorney who assists in this transaction with elder abuse.

2. Create an advance health care directive.

An advance health care directive, also known as a "living will," allows your physician, family, and friends to know your health care preferences, including the types of special treatment you do or do not want at the end of life, and your desire for diagnostic testing, surgical procedures, cardiopulmonary resuscitation, and organ donation. It also allows for an agent (someone you choose) to have authority to make decisions regarding artificial nutrition and hydration and any other measures that prolong life—or not. In essence, you are granting power of attorney for your health care needs, just as you have done for your financial matters. You can also outline your preferences about where you want to live if you need assistance with activities of daily living or skilled care.

I received a call from a man who was in a panic. He had brought his father, who was 78 and had dementia, to the emergency room because he had been vomiting all morning. He knew his father had an inherent distrust of the medical community, having been in medical sales his entire life. The ER doctor wanted to do a CT scan. The father objected. He wanted to go home. Because he had dementia, he became more and more irate at the doctor's suggestion that he was going to do a CT scan. "I want to go home with my son," he said. The doctor handcuffed this gentleman's wrists and ankle cuffed his legs to the gurney and whisked him off for the test, while his son stood by helpless—powerless.

Shortly after the scan, this gentleman was taken to a psychiatric ward at a hospital and placed on a three-day hold. In California this is called a 5150. In essence, under the state's Welfare and Institutions Code, if an officer, member of the attending staff of a hospital, or professional person has probable cause to believe that the person is, as a result of a mental disorder, a danger to others or to himself or herself, or gravely disabled, he can be transported against his will to a designated psychiatric inpatient facility for evaluation and treatment for up to 72 hours. I was called when the hospital decided to add another 14 days to the hold. Why? Because when they cuffed his ankles, they cut his thin skin and caused a MRSA infection. Of course, they never paid much attention to the oozing on his ankles until they were blistering red.

The first question I asked the son was whether there was an advance health care directive. Had he been his agent, his father could have gone home with him, would not have had any tests, and would not have suffered so.

This not-so-hypothetical scenario demonstrates that it is extremely important to have an advance health care directive and to choose an appropriate agent to carry out your wishes. If this is impossible, you can name a professional fiduciary. If you do not know one, ask your attorney or CPA for a referral to a reputable bank or professional.

Please make sure that if you list co-agents, they truly have the ability to carry out your wishes and can work in harmony with one another. Sometimes, one sibling will object to the prospect of withholding life sustaining support stating, "I know what mother would want here," even though her directive is clear. The other sibling, a strict constructionist, will re-articulate the words of the document in an effort to uphold what he thinks his mother meant. This could not only result in prolonging a situation that you do not desire, but it could break the family forever.

It is also important that you be cognizant of the tension that can be created by your choice of agent for finances if it is different from the choice you make for health care. For example—and these are scenarios that I see all of the time—let's suppose that you have become cognitively impaired to the point that your powers of attorney have sprung into effect. (Most powers of attorney are drafted this way, otherwise your agent could access your funds at any time for any reason.) The child that you chose as your agent for your health care directive has been caring for you, but your situation has become more chronic and she cannot afford to take any more time from her job or her family. Additionally, she is ill-equipped to handle your disease. She has the power to hire a caregiver or place you into an environment that is better suited to help you.

Now, let's suppose that your son, the accountant, is the agent under your power of attorney for finances and he refuses to dole out the money for any of this because he is fiscally conservative, out of touch with your daughter's plight, or greedy (the cost of care is quite expensive). This stalemate can cause a host of problems. Your health will decline rapidly and the chances of you leaving this planet with dignity will begin to wane. Your daughter will become sick with worry and just plain sick from continuing on her caregiving path. Your children will cease to speak to one another upon your death.

There are other reasons to make sure that you assign an agent. For example, a recent study revealed that one-fifth of Medicare nursing home patients with advanced Alzheimer's or other dementias were sent to hospitals or other nursing homes for questionable reasons in their final months. These patients were more likely to be subjected to torturous and futile life extending interventions such as feeding tubes, time in intensive care in the last month of life, severe bedsores, or late enrollment in hospice (three days or less before death). According to that study, the most vulnerable were those **without advance health care directives**.

Medicaid pays, on average, $175 per day (depending on the state) for long-term care, but Medicare will pay *three times that for skilled nursing care* after a patient returns from three days or more in a hospital. The study provided no evidence that money motivated such transfers or that there was wrongdoing involved. However, there was a large variation in transfer rates from state to state, and this suggests that money may be playing a role.

If you have an advance health care directive in place you can state that you do not want to be hospitalized before a nursing home can make that decision. This way, your family and doctors can focus on comfort care rather than trying to prolong your life and torture you in the process. When the time comes, your family will be able to say, "This is what she (or he) wanted."

3. Tell your children where your important documents are located.

A sudden fall or an automobile accident can precipitate a deluge of anguished decisions and rapid changes requiring a sudden scramble to locate account numbers to pay bills while you are in the hospital. I have been called by scores of boomers tangling with issues like trying to figure out why a parent's insurance company is denying coverage for an X-ray or how to assess the most appro-

priate living situation for a parent in collaboration with a sibling
who lives three states away.

*I had a new client. She was the loveliest woman I had ever met.
One day, I received a series of calls from her neighbors and friends who
left messages that "Marilyn is going to die." They were frantic. She
would not let them take her to the hospital or to a doctor. She was
afraid to go down the stairs and was just stubborn. I canceled all of
my appointments, turned around on the freeway and spent the next
two hours convincing her to allow me to have a concierge doctor visit
her, and then finally convinced her to let me call 911. When they came
to get her I had to rummage through her belongings to find her insurance cards and medical records, which I had indicated in my initial
opinion letter she needed to organize. The fire captain would not leave
the scene without these documents. It took me 15 minutes. This could
have meant the difference between life and death.*

It is important for your children to know where your Social
Security and Medicare cards are. If you have a Medicare supplement or if you are in a Medicare Advantage plan, or if you have
secondary insurance, they need to know this and they need to
know where to find all of the related documentation. If you served
in a war, you may be entitled to veterans' benefits; you should
share your identification number with your children. If you have
long-term care insurance, direct them to the policy.

If your child is the trustee of your revocable trust and your
assets are in that trust, you also need to share that document with
her. Even if you do not want your child to see the substance of
this document, *you must provide it to her.* If you do not, you will
not be able to afford the care you need. If this is a problem, please
name someone else to be the trustee.

I'll be honest; I have really never liked filling out the emergency
card for my kids' school, but I do it every year. The school needs
to know who to call in an emergency and who my children's pedi-

atrician is. They need to know what insurance we carry. I dreaded this beginning of the year paperwork, failing to see the need for so much information, and I fought it at every touch of the pen to the card. But when my daughter was rushed to the hospital twice last October because she had two unprovoked seizures, I got it. The school reached our pediatrician and me instantly and the ambulance was able to get her to the hospital where the admission process went smoothly. If the school did not collect all of this information, my daughter would have suffered. Likewise, if you don't share, you will suffer. If you feel overwhelmed by this task, you can download my book of essential forms by going to my website, www.susanbgeffen.com.

If you are reading this book, and if you love your children, please talk to them. If they will be there to catch you when you fall, ***it is their damned business***. You might think that you do not want to be a burden to your children. You may have even articulated this loud and clear. But those are just thoughts and words that have no feet. The burden is created when your children do not have what they need to make sure you are cared for.

Regardless of the theory to which you subscribe, one thing is evident—we have the power and opportunity to effect meaningful change. Our future is not a paint-by-number set, but rather a blank canvas. We have the power to choose whether the painting we collectively create will be rich in color like those of the Romantic Movement, inspired by imagination, independence, and autonomy. The passion of these artists was fueled by a revolt against the strict rules of classicism. For those of you who are older, born before the baby boom, it is not too late to plan for your future. As long as you are alive, you have a future. Don't let anyone convince you otherwise. You are not an object—an old person—you are a beautiful cellular miracle evolving though time. We should all be inspired to revolt. It's like the Beatles said, "I am he as you are he as you are me and we are all together."

CHAPTER 2

I Will Shoot Myself If I Ever Have to Go into a Nursing Home

People often utter, "I will shoot myself if I have to go into a nursing home," and a friend of mine, Steve Moses, Director of the Center for Long-Term Care Reform, responds, "That's assuming that you remember where you put the gun." I actually had a woman tell me that if it came down to being placed in a nursing home, she would jump into the pool in her backyard because she did not know how to swim. After wondering why she had a pool in her backyard to begin with, I thought to myself, "That assumes you will remember where it is." I think that you get the message. These are really stupid things to say.

So many of the people I meet with speak and live in this land of theory. They fail to understand that 50 percent of people over 85 years of age will get Alzheimer's disease.[11] This is a cognition stripper that deprives its victims of the privilege to make choices about their fates, including death by self-inflicted means. With your free will and mental capacity gone, it is likely that you will be *placed* in a nursing home by a loved one or a court imposed conservator.

Your placement will not be for lack of love. It will be because those you love are ill-equipped to care for you. It will be because when you were lucid, you proclaimed that you did not want to "be a burden to your children," but you failed to make a plan to ensure that your feet matched your words. It is this mistake of speaking in theory that thrusts families into panic mode and forces unpalatable decisions upon them.

In this chapter, I will tell you what a nursing home is, how nursing homes evolved in this country, how they are reimbursed, and what the future looks like for these facilities. Once you have a better understanding of what it means to be in a nursing home, I am certain you will also understand why it is so important that you plan carefully to avoid them.

What Is a Nursing Facility?

Nursing homes, nursing centers, convalescent homes, convalariums, sanitariums, or skilled nursing facilities. These are all different names for nursing facilities. Residents of nursing facilities often cannot walk and generally need help performing at least one activity of daily living (feeding, dressing, toileting, bathing, etc.). They also may have substantial memory loss. Skilled nursing facilities are intended for individuals who require an extremely high degree of ongoing personal care, such as individuals in late or final stage dementia, those who need a period of rehabilitation and therapy following an injury or hospitalization, or others who need specific medical care that cannot be performed in an assisted living setting. Many times people who have no personal financial resources and who qualify for Medicaid enter skilled nursing facilities rather than assisted living care homes, which (with limited exceptions) can only be paid for privately.

The staff of nursing facilities includes registered nurses, licensed nurses, and certified nursing assistants. Nursing facilities must have easy access to doctors. All nursing homes must be licensed by the state in which they operate and are required to comply with rigid standards enforced by regular facility inspections and extensive evaluations. Each state inspects nursing homes to assess compliance with federal standards for adequacy of staffing, quality of care, and cleanliness of facilities. These inspection results are technical in nature and are therefore sometimes difficult for consumers to interpret. The history and logistics of the survey system and the relatively new Five-Star rating system for consumers will be explored in later chapters.

According to the U.S. Bureau of the Census, slightly over 5 percent of people aged 65 and older occupy nursing, congregate care, assisted living, and board-and-care homes; about 4.2 percent are in nursing homes at any given time. The rate of nursing home use increases with age, from 1.4 percent of the young-old (ages 65–74) to 24.5 percent of the oldest-old (ages 85+). Almost 50 percent of those 95 and older live in nursing homes, and these individuals have an average life expectancy of approximately six months once they arrive.[12] Should I fail to persuade the estimated 78 million baby boomers to take action, an equal proportion (5 percent, or 3 million) of you are destined for these facilities.

How Did Nursing Homes Evolve? (Or, should I say, have they?)

In order to understand where the nursing home industry is headed, we should consider from whence it came. Prior to the industrial revolution, older relatives lived with extended family, which was conducive to an agrarian lifestyle. There was a lot of space for extended families to live with one another and much work for the aged individual in rural settings, assuring continued productivity.[13] Family roles were well defined. Men and children worked in fields; women, as their gender roles demanded, worked in the home.[14]

With the American Industrial Revolution, there was a rapid shift away from more localized family-based agrarian or small business enterprises to those that required longer hours, often away from immediate family, and work that was not of immediate importance to the family itself. Women had opportunities outside the home. This period had a profound effect on socioeconomic and cultural conditions. As the Industrial Revolution brought more people to cities, families spread out and often people had no local extended family to fall back upon when they were in need. Urbanization displaced families and changed how they interacted with one another.[15]

With new employment opportunities opening up for women, men, and children in New England and across America, families were now more free to split apart, move away, or engage in work that their genders or ages might not have previously allowed. It was during this period that divorce rates began to increase.[16] The result was a growing number of single and widowed people who had no one to take care of them in their old age. With no family to live with and no daughters at home to care for them, older adults were increasingly placed in facilities coined "poor houses" or "almshouses," which were often viewed as dumping grounds for the poor and elderly. Placed alongside the insane, the inebriated, or the homeless, the elderly were simply categorized as part of the community's most needy recipients.[17]

The first homes for the elderly were established by churches and women's groups and catered to widows and single women with limited resources. Homes such as the Indigent Widows' and Single Women's Society in Philadelphia and the Home for Aged

Women in Boston were a far better option than had previously been available. Advocates for these asylums contrasted their benevolent care with the horrors of the almshouses, but high entrance fees and requests for certificates of good character belied this perceived altruism. These requirements worked to shut out the neediest, who had no choice but to reside in the almshouses.

By the beginning of the twentieth century, sensibilities about caring for the poor and incapacitated had begun to change. Specialized facilities were built for children, the mentally ill, and younger infirm individuals, but little was done for the elderly. As younger indigents were transferred to institutions tailored to their specific needs—such as orphanages, work homes, hospitals, or insane asylums—elderly residents simply became a bigger percentage of the almshouse population. In 1880, one-third of the residents of almshouses in the United States were elderly; by 1923, two-thirds were elderly—an increase of 76 percent.

In response to these changes, the names of asylums were altered. For example, in 1903, the New York City Charity Board renamed its public almshouse the Home for the Aged and Infirm. The City of Charleston followed suit in 1913, transforming their almshouse into the Charleston Home. In these institutions, their managers claimed, the old could find everything they needed in their last days. But the reality of these name changes was much like Shakespeare's line in Romeo and Juliet: "What's in a name? That which we call a rose by any other name would smell as sweet." It is rumored that Shakespeare was alluding to his competitor, the Rose Theatre, with its smell and unsanitary conditions. Likewise, these were still almshouses. The homes were still horrible, still dirty and unsanitary. More importantly, there was much physical abuse and neglect in these settings.[18] By the 1930s, the tangible horrors of the almshouses and the rising percentage of aged individuals within such institutions convinced officials that radical measures needed to be taken.

In 1935, the Social Security Act was signed into existence by President Franklin Delano Roosevelt. Social Security was made universal, rather than needs-based. The federal government matched grants to each state for Old-Age Assistance. Now people could live in private care facilities or in their homes and still collect the Old-Age Assistance payments. Because of the continued stigma attached to the almshouses, however, those in public housing did not receive pension payments.

This proviso was essential for establishing both the popularity and legitimacy of the Social Security legislation. In asserting the constitutionality of the Social Security Act (1935), Supreme Court Justice Benjamin Cardozo, writing for the majority, proclaimed, "the hope behind this statute is to save men and women from the rigors of the poorhouse as well as the haunting fear that such a lot awaits them when the journey's end is near."[19]

The attempt to eradicate almshouses through pension legislation had unforeseen consequences. Excluding those in public housing from pension benefits proved to be disastrous to the frail and marginalized population of older adults. While intended to discourage almshouse living, pension advocates had overestimated the impact of pensions on the lives of the needy elderly. Their assumption that individuals could live independently (outside the almshouses) with monthly annuities was faulty because most of the residents were infirm and sick, with various ailments that required nursing or medical care in some type of institution.

The fact that almshouse inmates were precluded from receiving payments contributed to the creation of more *unregulated* private old-age homes, as older adults who needed long-term care were forced to seek shelter in unregulated sanitariums. In some cases, such a move was more a change in name than in place. In Kansas, for example, immediately following the enactment of Social Security, officials transferred well-established county homes into private control, although neither the residence nor its supervisors changed. Classifying the residents as recipients of private care enabled the institutions to receive the residents' monthly annuities.

All of this changed in the 1950s, when the Social Security Act stipulated that states needed to establish some form of licensing for nursing homes. By this time, the will of policymakers to obliterate the much reviled almshouses had clearly succeeded. The majority of poorhouses had vanished from the backdrop of age-centered care, unable to thrive once their residents no longer received federal annuities. Consequently, and partly attributable to the lobbying of public hospital associations, Congress amended Social Security to allow federal support to individuals in public facilities. Moreover, new legislation, including the Medical Facilities Survey and Construction Act of 1954, allowed for the development of public institutions for the neediest older adults. Now, both public and private nursing home residents were granted federal support for their assistance and older adults could obtain the long-term care that their conditions warranted.

From this grew federal regulations, including Congress' enactment of Medicare and Medicaid in 1965, which brought both financial aid and protection to the elderly living in nursing homes.[20] Specifically, Medicare and Medicaid spawned an increase in federal funding of nursing homes and provided additional impetus to the growth of the nursing home industry. Between 1960 and 1976, the number of nursing homes grew by almost 150 percent, nursing home beds increased by over 300 percent, and the revenues received by the industry rose 2,000 percent. Much of this growth was spawned by private industry: By 1979, at least 79 percent of all institutionalized elderly persons resided in commercially run homes.[21]

Investigations of the industry in the 1970s revealed that a good number of nursing homes provided substandard care. They were called "warehouses" for the old and "junkyards" for the dying by numerous critics. The majority of them, proclaimed Representative David Pryor in his attempt to initiate legislative reform in 1970, were "halfway houses between society and the cemetery."[22] As a result, policymakers began to enact numerous government regulations in order to control the quality of long-term care. Specifically, in 1971, the Office of Nursing Home Affairs was created to oversee a myriad of agencies responsible for nursing home standards. Shortly thereafter, in 1972, Social Security reforms established one set of requirements for facilities supported by Medicare and for skilled-nursing homes that received Medicaid.

In 1983, The Health Care and Financing Administration (HCFA)—what we now call the Centers for Medicare and Medicaid Services (CMS)—contracted with the Institute of Medicine (IOM) to conduct a study on nursing home care in America. HCFA was concerned that nursing homes were not providing a sufficient level of care and that the enforcement system was too lax. As a result, IOM published its report in 1986, titled "Improving the Quality of Care in Nursing Homes."[23]

In 1987, the United States Department of Health, Education and Welfare established health and safety standards for nursing homes wishing to participate in federally funded programs.[24] These standards subjected nursing homes that received Medicare and Medicaid to minimum federal quality standards promulgated by the HCFA. The Omnibus Budget Reconciliation Act of 1987 (OBRA-87) required all nursing homes receiving Medicare and Medicaid funds to comply with over 100 new quality standards.[25] Specifically, it still mandates that facilities provide each patient with the care that will enable him or her to "attain or maintain the highest practicable physical, mental and psychological well being." Additionally, it mandates that nursing homes provide around the clock care to residents and be staffed by licensed practical nurses, with a minimum of one registered nurse for an eight hour period each day.

To monitor compliance with these conditions, nursing homes must enter into provider agreements that permit unannounced annual standard surveys.[26] State surveyors, pursuant to a contract with the Department of Health and Human Services, conduct annual surveys of nursing homes that receive Medicare and Medicaid payments in order to determine whether they are in substantial compliance with the participation requirements.[27] Nursing home residents and their families are thus able to voice institutional complaints to ombudsmen—paid employees and unpaid volunteers who receive and handle suspected allegations of nursing home abuse. In 1997, 880 paid employees and 6,800 certified volunteers handled 191,000 complaints and shared information with 201,000 citizens.[28]

As will be further explored in later chapters, these policies have failed to uniformly raise the standards of all nursing homes. Arguably, these attempts by the legislature to control nursing homes with the promise of federal funds have had limited impact on the problems that plague long-term care for older adults. Nevertheless, nursing home care is still a reality for many of the nation's oldest old and poor. As of 2000, nursing homes have become a $100 billion industry, paid largely by Medicaid, Medicare, and out-of-pocket expenses. Most importantly, we have not progressed very far in the treatment of our elderly.

A separate but related issue has to do with the fact that mental illness is one, and sometimes *the* decisive factor contributing to placement in a nursing home.[29] Currently, more than 500,000 people with mental illnesses (excluding dementia) reside in U.S.

nursing homes on any given day, greatly exceeding the number in all other health care institutions combined.[30] Importantly, many of these individuals are below the age of 65—according to a 2011 study, many Medicaid beneficiaries aged 22 to 64 with serious mental illness are admitted to nursing facilities rather than to psychiatric facilities. In fact, the Associated Press has reported a national trend toward placing younger, physically able people with mental illness in nursing homes; as of 2009, this population now makes up 9 percent of the nation's nearly 1.4 million nursing home residents, up from 6 percent in 2002.[31] Nearly 16 percent of nursing home residents aged 22 to 64 had diagnosed mental disorders, while 45.5 percent received antipsychotic medication.[32] This trend, together with the problems of monitoring and compliance that I will explore in more detail later in the book, surely pose a risk to older, frailer residents. Before I explore those issues, it will first be helpful for you to understand a bit more about how nursing homes operate.

CHAPTER 3

Investigators, Surveyors, and Citations, Oh My!

Before I take you to the edge of what I like to call statistic saturation syndrome, I need to first explain more about how nursing homes are reimbursed by the government and how they are evaluated. Taking the time to understand this will help you if you have to search for a home. Likewise, if you want to get more involved in the political process as an advocate for change, you will need to know how the Centers for Medicare and Medicaid Services (CMS) operate. Most importantly, it will enable you to understand the statistics that I cite. For example, when you read that in 2004, 15.61 percent of facilities received deficiencies for inadequate infection control, and that this rose to 30.43 percent by 2009, you will be able to visualize how those statistics were derived and who shoulders their consequences. Here it goes.

Medicare and Medicaid: A Primer

First, it is critical for you to have a basic understanding of Medicare and Medicaid, both of which are important in understanding how nursing homes get paid. **Medicare** is the federal health insurance plan for all eligible individuals age 65 and older. Because of its universal availability, almost everyone over age 65 in this country is covered by Medicare. There are currently about 40 million Medicare beneficiaries nationwide. **Medicaid** is a means-based assistance program available to low income people, regardless of age. It is run by state and local governments within guidelines set by the federal government, and it therefore varies by location.

There are a lot of people who think Medicare pays for long-term care in a facility. In fact, Medicare coverage is provided only if you require doctor-ordered daily skilled nursing care or physical, occupational, or speech therapy on a daily basis. Nursing home care is limited to 100 days per spell of illness, which begins with the first day of inpatient care in a hospital or nursing home and ends when you have been hospital- and nursing home-free for 60 consecutive days.

The benefits vary across these 100 days. Specifically, Medicare will fully pay for the first 20 days of a skilled nursing care facility as long as you were receiving inpatient services in the hospital for at least three full days within 30 days of entering the facility. The next 80 days are also covered, but there is a $144.50 per day co-payment. Many people purchase Medicare supplemental coverage to take care of this and other relevant deductibles.

There is a misconception that Medicare *automatically* covers up to 100 days of all nursing home stays. In actuality, 100 full days of Medicare coverage are not that likely. Not all nursing home admissions come from a hospital (a prerequisite for Medicare coverage). Also, a hospital stay resulting in nursing home care does not automatically qualify for Medicare coverage, since the stay may have been less than three full days or there may not be a need for skilled care. Therefore, it is likely to be for much less than 100 days.

I have had several clients confused about the inpatient/outpatient distinction. Some had been in the hospital for over three days, but they were only being observed by a doctor to determine if they needed to be admitted as inpatients or discharged. But those three days did not count, even though they had spent three nights at the hospital.

I was especially frustrated by one call I received this year. A 94-year-old woman was discharged from a hospital within two days of breaking her pelvis. The discharge planner told her son (who signed the discharge papers without the legal authority to do so) that his mother would only need one week in a skilled nursing facility to rehabilitate. The facility subsequently told her that she would need to be there for at least a month. Because she had only had a two-day stay in the hospital, Medicare would not pay. She was left to figure out how to come up with $8,000 to cover the cost.

Medicaid will cover nursing home costs for individuals who meet the program's income requirements for as long as they require skilled care. The program covers almost half of all nursing home costs nationally, and it is the fifth largest expenditure for the federal government behind national debt, defense, Social Security, and Medicare. Federal Medicaid grants are growing so fast they will soon surpass Medicare spending. After applying state funds to federal matching funds, Medicaid is usually the biggest chunk of state budgets, following education. The General Accounting Office estimated that in 2004, 35 percent of Medicaid payments went for long-term care services. In 1998, Medicaid paid for 46.3 percent of the $88 billion received by all U.S. nursing homes. As of 2009, of the 1.4 million residents in nursing homes, 64 percent had their care paid by Medicaid, versus the 22 percent who paid for their care directly out of pocket or through private payers, such as through long-term care insurance.

As a means-based program, Medicaid will not pay for your stay at a nursing home unless your assets are below $2,000. I am sure that many of you have heard that you should spend your assets down in order to qualify. Some people just give their assets away and operate under the misguided assumption that the system allows this. I will discuss Medicaid qualification in a later chapter under financing, but at this point suffice it to say: DO NOT TRY THIS TRICK AT HOME.

How Are Nursing Homes Monitored?

Any nursing facility that receives reimbursement from Medicare and/or Medicaid must be certified as meeting certain federal requirements. So how does this work? The Centers for Medicare and Medicaid Services (CMS) contract with all of the states to perform routine surveys of nursing facilities. They must comply with rigid standards enforced by regular inspections and extensive evaluations to ensure that federal standards of care— such as adequacy of staffing, quality of care and cleanliness of facilities—are met. The results of these inspections are technical in nature and can be very difficult for consumers to interpret.

All nursing facilities must be inspected no less than once every 15 months, with a statewide average time between inspections of 12 months. In addition, CMS requires that at least 10 percent of inspections be "staggered" (i.e., started outside of normal business hours). Each state is responsible for keeping surveys unannounced and their timing unpredictable, giving the agency doing the surveying greater ability to obtain valid information. Federal regulations do not allow states to inspect nursing homes with "good" inspection records any less frequently than those with "bad" records. That would be like assuming my son would not sneak candy because he had one dentist appointment that did not result in a filling or tooth extraction.

A standard inspection consists of seven federally mandated steps. The federal *State Operations Manual* (*SOM*) sets forth the standards that inspectors must apply and the guidelines that help them apply those standards, both of which are complex. The *SOM* has hundreds of pages and contains 274 regulatory standards that nursing homes must meet at all times. The standards cover 16 different categories of operation, including administration, dietary services, infection control, life safety, physical environment, quality of care, quality of life, resident assessment, and resident rights. Deficiencies are identified when the statute or its regulations are violated; these violations are identified based on observations of the nursing home's performance or practices.

Some requirements must be met for each resident and any violation is considered a deficiency. For example, each resident must have a comprehensive care plan. Other requirements focus on facility systems and are evaluated comprehensively. For each deficiency, inspectors must use professional judgment to assess how many residents or staff are affected by or involved in the deficient practice (scope) and the amount of actual or potential discomfort or harm involved for residents (severity). These two determinations result in the inspection team assigning each deficiency a letter code to indicate scope (A through L, with level "A" deficiencies being the least serious) and a number code to indicate severity (1 through 4).

A level one deficiency has the potential to cause no more than a minor negative physical, mental, or psychosocial impact on a resident—for example, if a facility fails to post its inspection report. In contrast, a level four deficiency is an "immediate jeopardy" situation requiring immediate action in order to avoid or end serious injury, harm, impairment, or death to a resident. For example, if during an inspection a resident with Alzheimer's is found laying outside on the patio burning in the sun and marinating in her urine-soaked pants (which was the case with one home I toured), this would be evidence that the nursing home does not have a working system in place to monitor residents with dementia. In all likelihood, a level four deficiency would be issued. The table below summarizes the relationship between scope and severity of deficiencies.

Deficiency Scope and Severity Grid
Severity Scope

Severity	Isolated	Pattern	Widespread
Level 4: A situation that has caused or is likely to cause serious resident injury, harm, impairment, or death.	J	K	L
Level 3: A situation that has caused resident harm.	G	H	I
Level 2: A situation that has caused minimal discomfort to a resident OR has the potential to cause resident harm.	D	E	F
Level 1: A situation that has the potential of causing no more than minimal discomfort to a resident.	A	B	C

NOTE: Harm is defined as a situation that compromises a resident's ability to maintain or reach his or her highest practicable physical, mental, or psychosocial well being, as defined by an accurate and comprehensive assessment, care plan, and provision of services. A nursing home with one or more quality of life, quality of care, or resident behavior and facility practices deficiencies issued at level "F" or "H" or above (the shaded area of the grid) is considered to be providing "substandard" care to its residents.

SOURCE: James Nobles, *Nursing Home Inspections* (St. Paul, MN: Minnesota Office of the Legislative Auditor, 2005), p. 9.

Once the inspectors are satisfied that they have gathered enough information, they prepare a draft inspection report that discusses each violation (or deficiency). They then meet with nursing home personnel, interested residents, and family members to present the preliminary list of deficiencies. After the inspection team leaves the facility, they finalize the "Statement of Deficiencies" and submit it to the team's district supervisor, who is responsible for reviewing the document and submitting a final copy to the facility and CMS. When the state has cited deficiencies during the course of a survey, the survey agency may, as necessary, conduct a post-survey revisit to determine if the facility now meets the requirements for participation.

When immediate jeopardy exists, the regional office or state Medicaid agency will impose termination and/or temporary management in as few as two calendar days (one of which must be a working day) after the survey that determined immediate jeopardy. In all cases of immediate jeopardy, the provider agreement must be terminated by CMS or the state agency no later than 23 calendar days from the last day of the survey if the immediate jeopardy is not removed. The regional office or state Medicaid agency may impose a civil money penalty between $3,050 and $10,000 per day of immediate jeopardy or a "per instance" civil money penalty from $1,000 to $10,000 for each deficiency.

Most states also conduct their own inspections using their own citation systems and can impose fines for the same violations. In California, for example, a state statute allows citations that impose a civil monetary penalty as Class B, A, or AA. The associated fines range from $100 to $1,000 for Class B, $5,000 to $20,000 for Class A and $25,000 to $100,000 for Class AA. The citation class and amount of the fine depend upon the significance and severity of the substantiated violation, as defined by California law. While states can impose these fines, they are more limited in their ability to effect change. Specifically, they can only recommend to CMS that a federal remedy other than a written plan of correction be imposed. CMS may impose, modify, or waive the state's recommended remedy.

Some criticize this system for the high degree of variation that arises from differences in how states determine specific deficiency citations and the different tags that are used to cite the same problem. Sometimes, differences in the number of deficiencies cited for a single problem of non-compliance also exist.[33] Even within a state, different branch offices can vary widely in their enforcement of the law. The concern is that this variation limits the usefulness of deficiency citations—not only for CMS but also for consumers and providers.[34] Nevertheless, at the moment, this is the system we are stuck with.

In the coming chapters, I will share more about how the evaluation system that I have just described can become one of several tools to help you find a good home. They *are* out there, especially if you assure them that you will be able to pay privately. But before we get to the practicalities of searching, it is important that you understand *what* is out there. In other words, now that you understand how the process works, let's look at *how well* it works. With that absolutely boring dissertation behind us, let's move on to the statistics of abuse and neglect. These are not boring. They are downright disturbing. Again, I hope not to use these stories in vain. It is my intention to give meaning to the plight of those who have suffered.

As you read the next chapter, keep in mind that abuse and neglect significantly shorten older victims' lives, even when the abuse and neglect are perceived as minor. Seemingly trivial incidents can have a debilitating impact on an older victim, and a single episode of victimization can markedly change the life of an otherwise productive, self-sufficient person. Older victims do not typically have the same support systems and reserves (physical, psychological, or economic) that they once had to fall back on. This magnifies each event, and even a single incident of mistreatment can trigger a downward spiral, leading to loss of independence, serious complicating illness, and even death.[35]

CHAPTER 4

Are You Kidding Me with These Statistics?

In perhaps one of the best-known court cases related to nursing home neglect, a malnourished, dehydrated, anemic elderly man was admitted to the hospital from Tucker House, a Pennsylvania nursing home. He was in severe pain, and had approximately 26 stage IV decubitus ulcers, one of which was the size of a grapefruit and to the bone. Another was so bad that it decimated his shoulder. He also suffered from a gangrenous leg with toes that were in the process of falling off. Troubled by what they saw, the emergency room staff called the Long-Term Care Ombudsman, who in turn contacted the state's attorney general. Ultimately, the United States Attorney investigated the matter and found that Tucker House had failed to provide the basic care required by law and regulation, not just to the resident who sparked the investigation, but to *other* residents who also died from unnecessary pressure sores, weight loss, malnutrition, and out-of-control

blood sugars. This systemic failure spawned an expanded investigation to other facilities owned by the same company, Geri-Med,
a chain with a history of non-compliance.

An Administration on Aging (AOA) study concluded that
"for every abused and/or neglected elder reported to and
substantiated by Adult Protective Services (APS), there are over
five abused and/or neglected elders that are not reported."[36]
Because victims are often reluctant to reveal abuse due to shame,
self-blame, denial, fear of reprisal, or desire for privacy,[37] many
assume that this AOA study actually *underestimates* the amount
of underreporting.[38]

If I were impressed with nursing homes in our country, I
would not be writing this book. If you want to know the truth
about whether or not there is widespread abuse and neglect in
nursing homes, you have turned to the right page. I did not
contrive the statistics that follow—nor could I. Because I was
absolutely so disturbed by the subject, I lost two sets of finger
nails in my graduate level statistics class and cried like a baby to
the teacher's assistants, twenty years my junior. I am just the
messenger. These are scary statistics. Remember, however, that by
the time you finish this book you will not be part of these statistics, because I will give you achievable alternatives.

With all of the regulations I described in the previous chapter,
you might assume that the frailest members of our community
are now safe from abuse and neglect. Don't be fooled. Statistics
do not lie. There are those who toe the industry line and criticize
the underlying mechanisms from which the statistics are derived.
However, consumers do not listen to academic deconstructions of
studies. Most people do not even vote. As a *consumer*, when I hear
that two weeks ago two women died from neglect at two different
facilities within 20 miles of my home, I am not concerned with
statistics or methodological weaknesses; I am concerned with

human suffering. As a consumer, the end result is all I need to hear. In our world, perception is reality. If the industry does not like our perception of it, it should stop neglecting its residents.

First, Let's Kill All the Lawyers

In recent years, the nursing home industry has been in financial straits, with the majority of the largest chains and many smaller entities forced to file for bankruptcy. The reasons for the financial crisis are in dispute.[39] The industry blames lawsuits and corresponding colossal judgments for their inability to provide quality care. The argument goes that if it were not for blood-sucking lawyers, the homes would have more money to provide care to their residents. I will get a lot of backlash from writing this but the truth is that according to a 2004 Harvard School of Public Health study of 27 nursing home attorneys (representing plaintiffs as well as long-term care facilities), nursing home litigation *is* a growing industry—but it is relegated to only a few jurisdictions.

Big lawsuits *are not* a national phenomenon. According to the Harvard study, three out of four dollars paid out by nursing home cases went to claimants in Florida and Texas.[40] These two states—together with California—are generally referred to as jurisdictional hot spots.[41] The confined nature of this litigation is further borne out by an analysis of data compiled by the Association of Trial Lawyers of America (ATLA); from 1986 to 2004, only 27 nursing home cases nationwide included an award for non-economic damages.[42] Most of these were in states considered "cold spots," such as New Mexico, without a single verdict in almost two decades.

There exists no national verdict reporting system, and little empirical data have been collected on the incidence of nursing home litigation or on the conditions that lead to these types of lawsuits. Professor Michael Rustad at Suffolk University Law

School has compiled the largest sample of nursing home verdicts to date. His study, reported in the 2006 *Elder Law Journal*, includes the vast majority of awards in the aforementioned hot spots. His analysis of *Jury Verdict Reporters* reveals 383 cases filed between 1990 and 2004: 77 in California, 178 in Florida and 128 in Texas. There were, however, only 186 plaintiffs' verdicts. The California sample revealed an average of approximately one plaintiff's verdict per year over this 15-year period. There was an average of two verdicts in Texas per year (35 cases total) and an average of slightly more than four per year in Florida.[43] Does this lack of verdicts in favor of plaintiffs mean that nursing homes don't warrant the knee-jerk negative reaction we all tend to have when we speak of them? Or is something else at play?

To support his contention that there are actually *too few* negligence and abuse cases, Rustad references the facility deficiency statistics of these three hot spot states in contrast to the lawsuits filed. In Texas, where there have been only 35 nursing home negligence verdicts over the last 15 years, 86 percent of nursing homes had *substantial deficiencies* that posed potential or actual harm to vulnerable nursing home residents; 94 percent of nursing homes failed to comply with HHS minimum staffing levels and nearly 40 percent of the violations were so serious that they posed risk of imminent death or serious injury to residents.[44] And in California, a 2003 United States House of Representatives committee study uncovered systemic neglect and abuse in California nursing homes; of 439 homes in Los Angeles County, less than 3 percent were in full, substantial compliance with federal standards.[45]

There is also support for this proposition in Florida, where one in four nursing homes failed to meet minimum quality standards between 1997 and 1998. A 2001 Florida Task Force study that examined claims in residents' rights lawsuits against nursing homes in Hillsborough County, Florida, supports Rustad's conclusion.[46] Of the 225 cases for which court files were available, not one seemed to meet the legal definition of "frivolous," or was devoid of merit. The primary cause of action in all the cases was the right to receive "adequate and appropriate health care." (The analysis included lawsuits brought under residents' rights statutes only.) Virtually all of the cases (95 percent) involved one or more of the following harmful incidents: pressure sores, falls, dehydration and malnutrition, or weight loss. Case details were not disclosed, because 98 to 99 percent of them were settled out of court.

The *Sun-Sentinel* and *Orlando Sentinel* reviewed 924 lawsuits filed against nursing homes in south and central Florida over a five-year period and similarly concluded "the vast majority of the lawsuits (alleging rape, physically abusive staff, poor medical decisions, or neglect) are anything but frivolous."[47] Almost half of the 924 lawsuits involved a resident's death; half alleged bedsores; one-third claimed infections; and one-quarter mentioned falls. Many of the suits accused nursing homes of causing more than a single injury to a patient.

An analysis of the content of the data set, an examination of *Verdict Search* and newspaper accounts, as well as interviews with ATLA attorneys, illuminate the factual circumstances leading to pecuniary and non-economic damages. According to Rustad, they "evoke surrealistic portrayals of abuse and mistreatment" and pervasive patterns of tremendous suffering such as cases where damages were awarded for, among other things, sexual assault, wrongful death, drowning of a dementia patient, and sepsis resulting in gangrene as a result of a patient being left to lie in her own feces.[48] Rustad concluded that nursing home litigation is neither frivolous nor on the rise, but rather is a by-product of substandard care, which often goes unreported.[49] Indeed, elder abuse is one of the most under-diagnosed and under-reported problems in the United States. Official prevalence and incidence statistics do not exist at a national level, state statistics vary widely, and there is no uniform reporting system.[50]

But let's get back to the claim that lawsuits are driving up the costs of long-term care. The California Advocates for Nursing Home Reform (CANHR) is a statewide, nonprofit advocacy organization dedicated to improving choices, care, and quality of life for California's long-term care consumers. In 2003, over the course of nine months, CANHR studied elder abuse litigation against 577 skilled nursing facilities housing 50 percent of the beds in California. It was the first comprehensive study of lawsuits filed against nursing homes in California.[51] The study came in direct response to a claim by the American Health Care Association (AHCA)—a nursing home trade association that primarily represents for-profit nursing homes—that the Elder Abuse and Dependent Adult Civil Protection Act (EADACPA) of 1991 had resulted in "thousands" of elder abuse complaints against long-term care providers, resulting in an insurance crisis. To support its claim, ACHA cited a series of studies conducted by AON Risk Insurance, consultants for AHCA.

Claims of an insurance crisis by these stakeholders persist, even though an AARP study attributes the cost and availability of nursing home liability insurance to multiple factors including, but not limited to, the property/casualty insurance cycle; premium cuts during the 1990s; and lower returns on investment income.[52] Likewise, an Americans for Insurance Reform study found that over the past 30 years, insurance rate increases were attributable to the ups and downs of the economy, *not* lawsuit payouts.[53]

The CANHR study was a comprehensive review of California Supreme Court civil indexes in counties that represented approximately half of all nursing home beds in the state. Like the Rustad study, a substantive review of the types of allegations emanating from these complaints paints a picture of egregious conduct by a few bad apples contaminating the barrel; 23 percent of the facilities accounted for more than 71 percent of the lawsuits filed. In these cases, damages were sought for wrongful death (representing 50 percent of the claims), untreated bedsores, amputations, dehydration, malnutrition, infections, falls, and physical abuse.

CANHR also found that the facilities with the highest number of lawsuits filed against them had been more frequently cited for deficiencies and received more consumer complaints than facilities that were not sued. Skilled nursing facilities with at least one lawsuit had approximately 85 percent more complaints and several times the rate of an "imminent danger of death citations" as facilities with no identified lawsuits during the same period. They also showed 45 percent more deficiencies cited by state inspectors.

These statistics are not a relic of a bad system that has since been improved. A 2010 report by the University of California, San Francisco shows trends in U.S. nursing homes by state for 2004 through 2009. The data are derived from the federal On-Line Survey and Certification System (OSCAR) reports of annual nursing home surveys by state licensing and certification programs for the U.S. Centers for Medicare and Medicaid Services. These statistics support the notion that there are some good facilities, but not enough. Across the country in a single year, about 156,000 deficiencies were issued to nursing homes for violations of federal regulations. In 2009, 24.7 percent of the nation's nursing facilities received deficiencies for poor quality of care, where facilities caused harm or jeopardy to residents. This was a 3 percent increase over 2004, indicating that there are still many quality problems in our nation's nursing homes.[54]

In December 2011, the California Department of Public Health ordered two Orange County assisted living facilities to pay fines over patient deaths involving "inadequate nursing care." At a Newport Beach nursing home, a female patient who needed assistance to use the toilet was left unsupervised and was found face down and without a pulse in the bathroom. The coroner determined her cause of death as spinal fracture caused by a fall. At another nursing home, a female patient died after a nursing assistant forgot to give her dentures so she could eat lunch. The patient, who had problems swallowing and chewing, was supposed to be given chopped meat. The woman was taken to the hospital after she was found blue in front of a ham sandwich that was partially eaten. At the hospital, a large piece of meat was removed from her throat. Less than a week later, she died from respiratory and cardiac arrest related to choking.

According to data from the CDC's National Center on Health Statistics, most of the deaths in nursing homes are caused by neglect traced to caregivers, on whom the elderly rely for food and liquid, and for turning them in their beds to prevent life-threatening sores. A national compilation of more than 500,000 nursing home deaths in 1999 lists starvation, dehydration, or bedsores as the cause on 4,138 death certificates. However, the number of such deaths "is much higher," according to investigators who compared nursing home patient medical records with their death certificates.[55]

If it were just greedy lawyers and not the despicable practices that many facilities allow, then why would the federal government, through the Department of Justice, use its limited resources to pursue cases of abuse and neglect? Recall that these facilities are subject to contractual promises to the federal government from whom they receive Medicare and Medicaid dollars. One of the many promises is to refrain from billing for non-existent goods or services. Hence there is a public health *and* fiscal interest in the pursuit of monetary damages by federal law enforcement.

The majority of the Department of Justice's cases to date that allege abuse and neglect in residential care settings (failures of basic care leading to profound malnutrition, dehydration, pressure ulcers, scalding, and other illness, injury, or death) have been pursued under the civil False Claims Act (FCA), a financial fraud statute.[56] Originally enacted after the Civil War to redress war profiteering, it is sometimes referred to as "Lincoln's Law," as it was passed at the urging of President Abraham Lincoln to combat the fraud being perpetrated on the Union by profiteers selling shoddy, defective, or nonexistent goods.[57] The Act provides a cause of action, treble damages, and penalties where a person (either an individual or entity) knowingly submits or causes to be submitted to the United States a false claim for payment.

The FCA has been the government's principal tool in fighting health care fraud. For the first time in 1996, and on several occasions since then, the United States pursued "failure of care" cases under the False Claims Act, where providers have used public funds but have failed to take care of residents in accordance with the standards specified by those programs. A failure of care case may be actionable under one or more of several alternative False Claims Act theories, including billing for nonexistent or worthless services, falsely certifying compliance with regulation and statutes governing care, or where there is a connection or nexus between poor care and conditions for repayment.

The first failure of care nursing home case pursued under the False Claims Act stemmed from the gross mistreatment of the man described at the start of this chapter. *United States v. GMS Management-Tucker, Inc., No. 96-1271* (E.D. Pa. Feb. 21, 1996), commonly known as the Geri-Med case, provides a great but sad example of how this statute works. When the tragedy of this man's situation came to light, there was no cognizable cause of action under state law to pursue the case.[58] When the United States Attorney ultimately investigated, the systemic failure they uncovered led to a larger investigation of other facilities owned by Geri-Med.

The investigation exposed significant failure of care problems with numerous facilities in the chain. The government sued, alleging that Tucker House submitted false claims for services that were alleged to be substandard. The United States retained several experts, including a geriatrician with expertise in nutrition and a decubitus ulcer specialist, in order to review various hospital and nursing home records. A review of the residents' records evidenced the fact that all victims suffered from a spiraling functional decline with inadequate provision of nutrients and that the residents became profoundly malnourished, thereby making it impossible for their bodies to heal the multiple decubitus ulcers that had developed. The inadequate provision of nutrition to the three residents occurred over a 15-month period of time.[59]

A settlement with the Office of Inspector General (OIG) of the Department of Health and Human Services (DHHS) was reached for $600,000 in False Claims Act damages. This represented monies received by the facility for the care of the residents who were harmed by their failures. Non-monetary relief was also ordered in the form of a consent judgment that put a monitor and protocols in place in Geri-Med facilities. These consent orders transcended remedying the treatment of the three victims who were the subject of the lawsuit by mandating the inclusion of all 18 facilities owned by Geri-Med (approximately 4,000 residents), including Tucker House. The orders also required the company to implement a state-of-the-art nutrition and wound care monitoring program at all of its facilities.

Another case, *United States v. Chester Care*, demonstrates the range of remedies available in the United States. A False Claims Act action was resolved in 1998, but the facility's abuse persisted after the settlement was reached—in other words, they just kept neglecting their residents. This spawned both a contempt action and a permissive exclusion action (the OIG has the authority to exclude every officer and managing employee of a sanctioned entity from even entering the facility). The OIG also ordered the assignment of a temporary manager and a temporary monitor to periodically inspect all of its facilities and to ensure the residents' safety.

The Department has pursued several more cases against long-term care facilities involving egregious failures of care with devastating consequences for the vulnerable victims. According to a recent study, between 1986 and 2001, the federal government recovered $8 for every $1 spent fighting health care fraud and abuse using the False Claims Act.[60]

It is true that there are significant potential fiscal and public health implications of recent bankruptcy actions, but when the industry blames its failure to care on the fact that there are too many regulations, it is like asking the public to accept rat droppings in its food because the restaurant industry must comply with oppressive health department regulations. Likewise, blaming the plaintiffs' bar is not only misplaced, but it is like saying that if personal injury attorneys did not file so many lawsuits, people would get into fewer accidents. Accidents may cause insurance rates to go up, but that is because of our collective driving habits.

In 1999, in the wake of the numerous bankruptcies of nursing home chains, CMS asked the state surveyors to conduct a survey of each facility owned by a bankrupt entity within 30 days of the bankruptcy filing, in order to ensure that the financial crisis did not have an immediate adverse effect on the residents.[61] Most importantly, where aggressive criminal prosecution of long-term care providers bankrupts a facility, divestiture and corporate integrity agreements as well as temporary independent monitors (paid for by the defendant) can be used to protect residents. A divestiture agreement forces a ne'er-do-well company to sell its properties (or have a court appointed trustee do so). These agreements promote the integrity of real people's housing and care, while ensuring that the vulnerable residents do not end up paying the price for the crimes of the facilities charged with their care. If these facilities go under *en masse*, we will truly be back to the days of the almshouses—or maybe, more optimistically, we will revert to a time when families lived together and cared for one another.

But If It's Not the Lawyers' Fault...

What follows are the real reasons there are a disproportionately small number of civil lawsuits and criminal prosecutions compared to the actual statistics of abuse and neglect:

Reason 1: Old People Are Not Worth Anything/Perceived Ageism

Despite OBRA-87 and the governmental studies that confirmed an epidemic of pain and suffering and widespread institutionalized neglect,[62] only a handful of civil lawsuits seeking financial penalties were filed against nursing facilities prior to 1990. Consequently, during this period, both insurers and nursing home providers enjoyed a relatively stable market for professional liability insurance.[63] While litigation is one way to supplement regulatory mechanisms and force change upon an industry, the plaintiffs' bar dismissed the possibility of filing nursing home negligence cases during this period because they believed "that the patients were too old and the damages too limited."[64]

Compared to a hospital patient, it is more difficult for a nursing home resident to sue. Most nursing home residents can not claim lost earnings, but many injured hospital patients can. Likewise, the reduction of an injured nursing home resident's life expectancy is typically small compared to that of a younger hospital patient with the same injury. Nursing homes do not perform hazardous operations, and proving a causal connection between a facility's conduct and a resident's death is difficult. Most nursing home residents are expected to die within a few years of entering a facility, so if a resident dies as a result of the facility's negligence, it is difficult to demonstrate that the death would not have occurred anyway.[65]

In the earlier years of their evolution, nursing homes were insulated from negligence or abuse litigation because most, as non-profits, were afforded charitable or governmental immunity. As more for-profit companies took over the industry, governmental immunity became less important and nursing home litigation slowly began to increase.[66] Simply stated, it was too difficult for nursing home residents and their families to sue and obtain compensation, even when substandard care caused death or serious injury to a resident.[67] *It did not mean that abuse was not widespread.*

Indeed, in a 1990 ground-breaking survey of nursing home personnel in one state, 36 percent of the nursing and aid staff reported that they had witnessed at least one incident of physical abuse during the preceding twelve months and 10 percent reported that they had themselves committed physical abuse.[68] The study also found that 81 percent of staff had observed—and 40 percent had engaged in—at least one incident of psychological abuse during the same 12-month period.

Arguably, any perceived rise in nursing home litigation must also be seen as a direct result of elder abuse statutes that established new remedies for abuse and neglect.[69] It is only recently that trial lawyers have begun to augment regulatory mechanisms by specializing in and litigating these cases.[70] Beginning in the early 1990s, nursing home neglect and abuse cases first arose as a legal specialty, and the number of claims has risen substantially since then.[71] Still, these cases were and remain few and far between because they are not sexy. We live in a youth-oriented and somewhat superficial world, and elderly victims may simply lack jury appeal.

Reason 2: Damage Caps/Codified Ageism

As I have already described, toward the end of the 1990s, there was a period of volatility in the nursing home liability insurance market that was blamed on an alleged increase in the number of lawsuits. This put greater focus on tort reform, a public policy response to cap non-economic damages (pain and suffering) in elder abuse cases.[72] The argument for caps on damages is premised on an assumption that legislative limits will lead to lower insurance premiums, which will in turn ensure quality health care. Yes, "the first thing we do, let's kill all the lawyers." This line was voiced by a barely recognizable character in Shakespeare's *Henry the Sixth* who believed that all lawyers do is shuffle parchments back and forth in a systematic attempt to ruin the common people.

As a lawyer, I feel compelled to come to the defense of my ilk. It seems as if my profession and the punitive damages that we seek are used as an excuse for things going awry in an industry, instead of the other way around. Punitive damages should cause change where massive failures in industries significantly harm humans. Can you imagine what would have happened if there was a cap on damages in the Ford Pinto exploding vehicle calamity?

In the first lawsuit involving a Pinto impact, the resultant fire killed two people. The jury awarded a very large verdict that was subsequently *reduced*. Things got significantly worse six months following that reduced verdict when there was another needless crash involving the Pinto, and this time three women were killed. This crash would not have happened if Ford had its bottom spanked hard enough the first time around. Following this crash, it was determined that the automobile's fuel system design contributed to the victims' deaths. The fact that Ford had chosen not to upgrade the fuel system design after the first two innocent humans were killed became an issue of public debate.

Perhaps if the verdict had not been reduced those women would still be alive. By conservative estimates, Pinto crashes caused between 500 and 900 burn deaths to people who would not have been seriously injured if their cars had not burst into flames. Burning Pintos became such an embarrassment to Ford that its advertising agency, J. Walter Thompson, dropped a line from the end of a radio spot that read "Pinto leaves you with that warm feeling." Ford waited eight years to fix the problem because its internal cost-benefit analysis, *which placed a dollar value on human life*, indicated that it wasn't profitable to make the changes sooner.

Ultimately, in February of 1978, a California jury created a nationwide sensation when it awarded the record-breaking sum of $128 million in a lawsuit stemming from the damage caused by the Pinto. Following the verdict, the Department of Transportation announced that the Pinto fuel system had a "safety related defect" and called for a recall. Ford agreed, and on June 9, 1978, the company recalled 1.5 million Pintos. Ford had no choice but to halt production of the car five months after the trial.

The Pinto example demonstrates how lawsuits can effect positive change by creating serious monetary consequences for companies that harm our fellow man. They can force not only those companies but also the market as a whole to take notice of the consequences of placing dangerous products on the market—or in the case of nursing homes, the consequences of not taking seriously the amount of abuse and neglect that they are responsible for.

Damage caps in nursing home cases relegate victims to economic damages or objective monetary losses like medical expenses or loss of employment and earnings. Elder victims are unlikely to have these types of damages; they do not suffer the loss of their professional lives and have no lost wages or self-financed medical bills. When such a cap was implemented in Texas in 2003, elder abuse attorneys took up other areas of practice; championing these causes was no longer financially feasible.[73] The figurative death of the lawyer was thereby accomplished. Also accomplished was the perpetuation of the notion that old people, which all of us hope to become, have no value.

Reason 3: They Have Hog Tied Us

According to an AARP representative who testified at the Joint Select Committee on Nursing Homes, a good majority of nursing home residents who have been injured due to a facility's negligence will never be compensated because many admission agreements include binding arbitration clauses with very low caps on damages, and these must be signed as a prerequisite to admission.[74] Citizens across the country are being forced into signing these documents in order to secure beds in nursing homes or in residential care facilities, or as a condition for adequate care. In so doing, they are surrendering basic constitutional rights and civil protections.

Facilities do this to prevent residents from being able to sue for abuse or neglect. When the document is signed, the resident loses the opportunity to have his grievances heard by a jury of his peers and to seek monetary compensation. The resident is deprived of any meaningful recourse if he is injured or his rights are violated. Nursing homes stack the deck in their own favor by explicitly limiting the time for response, selecting partial rather than impartial decision-makers, limiting discovery, and limiting statutory remedies, including damages. These agreements can dramatically curtail the amount of damages a plaintiff receives. The decision of an arbitrator is final and there is no appeal. These proceedings are not part of the public record and are not subject to judicial review. If you are researching a facility and do not uncover lawsuits against it, are you likely to operate under the misguided assumption that a facility has a good record of care? Not anymore; now you know.

Although they are not mandatory, arbitration agreements are seldom if ever negotiated at arm's length. The clause is typically buried in the middle of eight- to 10-page documents. Moreover, they are presented at an opportunistic time when the family is highly motivated to do everything necessary to ensure that their loved one receives urgent medical care. To that end, it is a "take-it-or-leave-it" proposition because there is no real choice when someone needs immediate care. Family members feel compelled to sign such agreements to ensure that the care of their family member is not compromised. In fact, if the agreement is not signed, the person probably won't be admitted to the facility in the first place.

Reason 4: The Shell Game

In response to lawsuits, some privately owned nursing homes have developed complex corporate structures that obscure who controls the facilities, making it difficult for attorneys to follow the money trail and collect damages. I myself experienced this confusion when I acted as in-house counsel for a large chain. Even as an attorney it was hard for me to unravel all of the players and their relationships to one another. According to an investigative article by Charles Duhigg of the *New York Times*, there is a maze of companies that protect profits and insulate owners from liability.[75] Sometimes owners and managers spread control of a facility among 15 companies and multiple layers of firms. As a result, it is very hard to definitively establish who is responsible for a resident's injuries, which hinders an attorney's efforts when a lawsuit is filed. If you really want to understand this byzantine structure, I urge you to read Charles Duhigg's article in its entirety.

This is not a partisan issue. Both Democrats and Republicans are in favor of stronger oversight and an investigation into why nursing homes bought by private investor groups scored poorly on 12 to 14 measures used to track long-term residents. In 2007, Senator Chuck Grassley [Rep] of Iowa forwarded two letters to the Government Accountability Office (GAO) asking it to examine how private equity ownership had affected the quality of care in nursing homes. In one of those letters, reprinted in the *New York Times*, Grassley questioned the legal schemes used by investment firms to shield them from liability, in effect denying both patients and family members any legal remedy against nursing homes. In Grassley's opinion, the use of such varied and complex ownership structures voided any transparency that would indicate who was responsible for resident care and the operation of investor-owned nursing homes.

Unfortunately, these tactics have served their purpose, dissuading lawyers from suing nursing homes. These structures of deception whereby hundreds of thousands of dollars are paid to management companies and affiliates to make it look like the operators are penniless when in fact they have simply diverted their rake, have stymied regulators as well. Even when they issue fines to investor-owned nursing homes, the penalties are difficult to trace and collect. Now, government programs require nursing homes to reveal when they pay affiliates so that the disbursements can be scrutinized; otherwise, it is a way for owners to pay themselves without revealing it.

Reason 5: Criminal Prosecution Obstacles

Much of the system meant to protect elders is drawn from the child protective services system.[76] Adult Protective Services (APS) provides social services to abused, neglected, or exploited older and/or disabled adults. APS is typically administered by local or state health, aging, or regulatory departments and includes a multi-disciplinary approach to helping victims of elder abuse. Services range from investigation of mistreatment to legal intervention through court orders or the appointment of surrogate decision makers such as legal guardians.

Federal laws on child abuse and domestic violence fund services and shelters for victims of these crimes, but there is no comparable federal law on elder abuse. The federal Older Americans Act (42 U.S.C. § 3001 et seq., as amended) does provide definitions of elder abuse and authorizes the use of federal funds for the National Center on Elder Abuse (NCEA) and for certain elder abuse awareness and coordination activities in states and local communities, but it does not fund adult protective services or shelters for abused older persons.[77]

Some states' APS laws only relate to individuals who reside in the community (what is called "domestic abuse"), while other APS laws also include individuals who reside in long-term care facilities (known as "institutional abuse"). States may define long-term care facilities differently, and some may also include other types of institutions (such as mental health facilities) in their statutes. In some states, APS investigates allegations of abuse, neglect, or exploitation against individuals who reside in the community—in residential settings, family members (including extended family) are responsible for committing almost 90 percent of elder abuse[78]—and a separate law addresses institutional abuse. There are also a few states in which there is no separate institutional abuse law, but the APS law provides that a state agency other than APS is responsible for receiving reports about and investigating institutional abuse.[79]

From an historical standpoint, law enforcement has rarely been involved in matters relating to abuse and neglect in long-term care. The Department of Justice has pursued some cases involving abuse and neglect in nursing homes, but there is no federal criminal abuse and neglect statute that makes failures of care actionable *per se*. An increasing number of states are passing laws that provide explicit criminal penalties for various forms of elder abuse. Legislatures are also signaling their intent that elder abuse be treated as a crime in other ways. For example, some Adult Protective Service laws include a provision stating that elder abuse may be prosecuted criminally, while others define certain acts (e.g., sexual abuse) in the same words or by reference to definitions that are used in criminal laws. Even if there is not a specific statute or provision authorizing criminal prosecution for elder abuse, a jurisdiction's basic criminal laws (e.g., battery, assault, theft, fraud, rape, manslaughter, or murder) can be used to prosecute someone who has committed an act of abuse against an older person. Some legislatures have enacted enhanced penalties for certain crimes against older persons.[80]

Here in California there are great, comprehensive laws about elder mistreatment. In Southern California, where I live, there are excellent resources for dealing with the complexities of elder abuse cases. Of particular note is the geriatrics program at the University of California, Irvine, which started the country's first Elder Abuse Forensic Center in May 2003.

Despite the plethora of statutory authority to do so, few criminal charges are filed. Take, for example, the case of Donald Mallory. Andrew Schneider and Phillip O'Connor published an article in the *St. Louis Post-Dispatch* in 2002 titled, "Nation's Nursing Homes are Quietly Killing Thousands." They discussed how thousands of elderly Americans have died due to neglect in nursing homes and they described Mr. Mallory's plight: He lost 40 pounds during a 37-day stay at a nursing home. Court records state that Mallory, 60, was dehydrated, malnourished and rife with infection from bedsores when he died. Doctors who reviewed his medical records for a lawsuit said neglect caused his death. The article also described the matter of Ruby Faye Martin, 88, who died of sepsis, an overwhelming bacterial infection that poisons the blood, at a Mt. Vernon, Illinois, nursing home. An evaluation of her medical records by a doctor who specializes in medical problems of the elderly stated that her death was caused or exacerbated by malnutrition and multiple infected bedsores caused by poor care at the nursing home.

Schneider and O'Connor exposed the fact that prosecutors charged no one in those cases, nor in the case of 57-year-old war veteran Rex Riggs, who was in stable condition when he was transferred to a nursing home. He was hospitalized with gangrenous infections that led to the surgical removal of his scrotum, penis and lower abdomen. He died three days later. Federal investigators said bad nursing care caused his death. Beyond these specific cases, the journalists examined the death certificates and the physicians' evaluations of 55 nursing home residents in Missouri and Illinois who had died in the previous two years and whose relatives decided to sue for neglect. The cause of death listed on the certificates in 42 of these cases differed from what the doctors said the actual medical records showed. According to the *Post-Dispatch* analysis of hundreds of these court cases across the nation, the vast majority of death certificates attributed the deaths to natural causes such as pneumonia, heart attack and—in some cases—"cessation of breathing," "heart stopped," "old age" or "body just quit."

To my knowledge, the first time federal criminal charges were filed was in a 2000 case that involved an elderly woman who wandered away from an Arkansas nursing home where she resided. She was found on the road outside the facility with a deep wound on her forehead as well as bruises and various other cuts.

The director of nursing (DON) and an aide returned her to the nursing home, where they changed her clothing and placed her in her bed before calling for an ambulance. The woman died within 24 hours, after having been returned to the facility by the hospital, which failed to take x-rays or perform a physical exam.

The DON lied to the hospital by telling them that the woman had fallen in her room and struck her forehead on a night stand. The lie was perpetuated by the DON and the facility's administrator over a four-year period to a myriad of law enforcement officials, including the Arkansas Long-Term Care Office, the FBI, and a state police detective. Ultimately, both pled guilty to making and conspiring to make false statements to federal officials regarding the events leading up to the resident's death under 18 U.S.C. Sections, 1001 and 1518, and they were each sentenced to 18 months imprisonment.[81]

For well over a year, ProPublica, along with other news organizations, scrutinized the nation's coroner and medical examiner offices, which are responsible for probing sudden and unusual fatalities. They found that the agencies "have sometimes helped to send innocent people to prison and allowed killers to walk free."[82] The story of a retired U.S. government scientist, Joseph Shepter, was at the center of this story. Mr. Shepter, who was paralyzed from a stroke and had dementia, spent two years living in a California nursing home. When he died, the nursing home's medical director stated that that his death was the result of heart failure brought on by clogged arteries. After he was buried, a tip from a nursing home employee prompted state officials to re-examine the case and reach a very different conclusion.

Mr. Shepter actually died of a combination of ailments often related to poor care, including an infected ulcer, pneumonia, dehydration and sepsis. His death was also hastened by the inappropriate administration of powerful antipsychotic drugs.

Initially, because he had been under a doctor's care, and that doctor classified his death as natural (not suspicious), a coroner investigation *was not* triggered. And because the doctor checked off a small box on the death certificate indicating that he never contacted the county coroner, there was no autopsy. There is an assumption by law enforcement that physicians report deaths accurately. In fact, in a great number of states, doctors are allowed to sign off on death certificates without having seen a patient in months or actually viewing the body. Hence, the reasons for Mr. Shepter's death went unchallenged.

Do you remember my hypothesis, "Old People Are Not Worth Anything?" How is this fact to support my theory? According to the Centers for Disease Control and Prevention, of the 1.8 million seniors who died in 2008, post-mortem exams were performed on just 2 percent. The rate is even lower—less than 1 percent—for elders who passed away in nursing homes or care facilities. It is hardly surprising, then, that since the story about Mr. Shepter first aired, ProPublica and *FRONTLINE* have identified more than three dozen cases in which the alleged neglect, abuse, or even murder of seniors got past authorities. If it were not for whistle-blowers, concerned relatives, and others, the truth about these deaths might never come to light.

Why aren't prosecutors filing criminal charges against nursing home employees who neglect patients? Is this not homicide? Does someone have to beat an elder in order to be punished for her death? Why does it seem like impunity is the impetus for the status quo? Some law enforcement officials with whom I spoke believe that such action should be classified as homicide. However, many prosecutors and district attorneys are reluctant to bring criminal charges against workers involved in preventable deaths because of the lack of evidence in such cases. Prosecutions are hampered by a number of variables, including the paucity of research developing forensic markers and methodologies to guide identification and diagnosis of abuse and neglect.

There is also a dearth of experts like forensic geriatricians or geriatric nurse practitioners who could provide assistance with investigation, consultation, and testimony. Further hindrances include the infrequent reporting and the rarity with which such cases are assigned priority and/or the necessary resources. Moreover, there is a lack of information about which measures are most effective in remedying existing abuse and neglect and in deterring and preventing future instances.[83]

The American Prosecutors Research Institute conducted interviews with elder abuse prosecutors and identified several barriers to prosecution:

> "The priorities in a prosecutor's office can change from elder abuse one day to gangs and drugs the next."
> "Training of the prosecutors is spotty at best. The training has to be ongoing and reflect the needs of the current staff in the positions."
> "Prosecutors will only take cases that they believe will result in conviction. These cases present complex issues and can be difficult to prove."
> "There is a lack of public education or public outreach on the topic from most prosecution offices."
> "There are systemic problems in the interplay between prosecutors, law enforcement, APS, nursing homes, and the roles each is to play."[84]

The fact that law enforcement is not currently playing a significant role should not be viewed as an indication that abuse rarely occurs in nursing homes or that reports of abuse are much ado about nothing. Based on the *persistent* reports of abuse and neglect, law enforcement should be playing a more significant role, and those who cause the abuse and neglect should be held responsible. But, again, the fact that it has not yet done so is a fortuitous anomaly.

A number of factors are now converging that may improve the outlook for elder abuse prosecution. Although the field is in its infancy in many regions, many law enforcement agencies are developing expertise in elder abuse; prosecutors have won high-profile cases in Washington, D.C. and other cities; law enforcement officers are becoming increasingly aware of the elder abuse problem and now have solid forensic studies upon which to rely.[85] All I can say to those who chide the statistics of abuse is, *Watch out.*

CHAPTER 5

Can Someone Help Me Out Here?

DRUM ROLL, PLEASE. NOW FOR THE BIGGEST PROBLEM WITH NURSING HOMES: They are woefully understaffed. I remember the days when I had four children all at once in this household. With my husband to help, there was a one to two ratio of parent to child. That was manageable, but difficult. While managing my baby, I had to ensure she would not fall to her death down our stairs or pick up a rogue object from the floor and place it in her mouth. When my husband was not here, I had to monitor what the older boys were doing on the Internet or what they were cooking in the kitchen. Mostly, I had to peel them off of one another. There was a cacophony of sounds to compete with as well. If I took my eye off any one of them I knew something bad could happen, including me losing my patience and abandoning any shreds of grace I had remaining. I knew when I was in trouble and I called my mother-in-law or a babysitter for help and relief. I never neglected them or beat them.

Let me be clear that I am not equating older adults to children; to do so would be to insult a cohort most deserving of our respect. Still, it is difficult to deny that the energy required to keep them safe and healthy is not dissimilar. I could no more leave my baby in a wet diaper without causing him to suffer a horrible rash or infection than an incontinent and immobile adult could be left in his diaper. I could not feed my baby carrots without expecting him to choke when he had only the ability to gum them. A facility cannot feed a resident with a swallowing disorder a huge piece of ham. I think you get the point. Some nursing home residents have to be very carefully watched and managed even if it means that the facility has to hire more help. These individuals are not babies, they are beautiful human beings with a lifetime of memories, hard work and wisdom behind them, but the fact is that they are dependent on others to watch over them. They would not be in nursing homes if that were not the case.

By now it should seem patently obvious that nursing home residents need special care. Yet, if there is a single thread running through most nursing home abuse cases, it is a lack of sufficient staff to take proper care of the residents.[86] It is widely believed that low nurse staffing levels are the strongest predictor of poor nursing home quality. Conversely, the highest-staffed nursing homes provide better care than all other homes.[87] Notwithstanding a uniform acceptance of this correlation, there is ample evidence to suggest that most facilities are plagued by understaffing.[88] In practical terms, this means that nurses and care providers are overworked. If staff cannot respond in a timely manner, mistakes happen. Pills are given too often or not at all; patient hygiene suffers; signs of serious illness are overlooked; residents fall and hit their heads on toilets and die.

In the case of Jack Evans, who lived at Potomac Nursing Center in Arlington, Virginia, the ramification of inadequate staffing was death *by neglect. Mr. Evans was partially paralyzed, could barely move, and had trouble breathing. Prior to his death, he would spend up to 12 hours a day in a wet diaper, unkempt and ungroomed. His widow, Mrs. Evans, also reported that his dentures were rarely removed, his finger-nails rarely cut, and that he went unshaved for weeks on end. Mrs. Evans would find his lunch still covered and untouched in the evening. She told news reporters that her husband could not feed himself, and often nobody would help him with the simple task of eating. He died of malnutrition. I could not have said it better than the attorney in that case who told a local news station: "If you're concerned about hiring another $10 an hour employee because you can't get to change a man's diapers more than once in 15 hours, that's where the poor nursing care comes in."*[89]

There are also concerns about the quality of the staff. Federal regulations prohibit Medicare and Medicaid nursing facilities from employing individuals who have been found guilty by a court of law of abusing, neglecting, or mistreating residents, or who have had a finding entered into the state nurse aide registry concerning abuse, neglect, or mistreatment of residents or misappropriation of their property. Yet, currently, only 43 states require nursing homes to run some kind of criminal background check on staff members, and only ten states (AK, AZ, DE, ID, MI, MS, NM, NV, NY, TN) require both a state and FBI background check that would detect convictions in multiple states. The requirements in these 10 states vary considerably in terms of what must be checked (e.g., statewide criminal history databases, publicly available sex offender registries) and who must be checked (e.g., direct-care workers only, all staff). Eight states (AL, CO, CT, HI, MT, ND, SD, WY) require no checks whatsoever.[90] Although the federal government has tried to streamline background checks through The Medicare Prescription Drug, Improvement, and Modernization Act of 2003 (also called the Medicare Modernization Act, or MMA) and The Patient Protection and Affordable Care Act of 2011, state participation is still *optional* and criminal background checks are left to the discretion of the states.

Common Problems in Nursing Home Care

There are a host of missteps that can result in neglect and serious injury—including death, as was the case in the two recent and unfortunate examples cited above—when there is not enough staff or when the staff has not been adequately screened. Some of the most common problems for which facilities are cited are outlined below. If these problems have been the subject of a facility's citations and have gone uncorrected by the facility, I would not give it a moment's consideration as a place for myself or a loved one.

Before I delve into the potential problems in nursing homes, it is worth demarcating the two distinct subgroups of residents in these facilities: those termed "short stayers," who are in the nursing home for convalescent or terminal care; and those termed "long stayers," who are using the nursing home as a long-term care facility.[91] While those simply rehabilitating and those residing in a nursing home are both susceptible to abuse, it is the older, more frail and vulnerable of the residents who are more likely to be endangered, as they can do little to assert their needs or complain if they are being mistreated. And if they have dementia or Alzheimer's disease, the situation can be even worse, as it may be difficult for family members to separate the truth of their accusations from the reality of delusions. My own Grandma Shirley had dementia and would consistently scream to us that the person giving her showers was beating her. Yet, there was no evidence to suggest that such was the case. Then again, I was only in my first year of law school and knew not of the horrors of this industry. I remain haunted by that.

Falls

Falls are the number one deficiency cited in the American Health Care Association's OSCAR report.[92] When a resident falls it is evidence of a "failure in accident environment." Forty-three percent of the facilities surveyed were deficient in this category. Between one-half and three-quarters of all nursing home residents fall each year.[93] That figure represents twice the rate of falls for older adults living in the broader community. About 1,800 of those who fall in nursing homes die each year from fall-related injuries. Those who survive frequently sustain hip fractures and head injuries that result in permanent disability and reduced quality of life.[94] Just the fear of falling can cause further loss of function, depression, feelings of helplessness, and social isolation.

Why does this come under the rubric of accident prevention? Environmental hazards in nursing homes cause 16–27 percent of falls among residents.[95] These hazards include wet floors, poor lighting, incorrect bed height, and improperly fitted or maintained wheelchairs.[96] As will be discussed next, the overuse of psychotropic drugs and sedatives can also increase the risk of falls and fall-related injuries.[97] During the three days following any change in these types of medications, fall risk is significantly elevated.[98] Other causes of falls include difficulty in moving from one place to another (for example, from the bed to a chair), poor foot care, poorly fitting shoes, and improper or incorrect use of walking aids.[99]

Professional Standards and Care Plans

The process of identifying a resident's abilities and needs is called an assessment. The plan describing how the nursing home will meet the resident's needs is called a care plan. Both assessment and care planning are critical to good nursing home care. The woman who choked on her sandwich was the unfortunate victim of a failure to either implement or follow professional standards or of a failure to implement or follow an appropriate care plan. She is not alone. According to the OSCAR report, these types of failures account for 34 percent and 29 percent of deficiencies, respectively. Federal law requires nursing homes to identify each resident's abilities and needs and to develop a plan to maximize their abilities and meet their needs.

In both of the cases cited, the residents had individual needs that required special attention. The respective nursing homes charged with their care should have developed written care plans to address these needs. Due to the large number of staff members, frequent turnover, and use of temporary staff members in many nursing homes, clearly written care plans are essential to ensure that the staff understands what each resident needs and how, when, and why the care is to be provided. Done properly, these evaluations improve the quality of care and quality of life in nursing homes. In these women's cases, there may have been care plans to address their challenges, but if there were, there was also clearly a failure to follow them.

Malnutrition and Dehydration

The levels of malnutrition and dehydration in some American nursing homes are similar to those found in many poverty-stricken developing countries where inadequate food intake is compounded by repeated infections.[100] Studies performed over the last five to 10 years using a variety of measurements of different nursing home subgroups have shown that from 35 to 85 percent of U.S. nursing home residents are malnourished. Thirty to 50 percent are substandard in body weight.[101] Malnutrition can happen for a variety of reasons. For example, difficulty with the mechanics of eating can be brought about by dental problems such as tooth loss or dentures that do not fit properly as well as mouth sores and swallowing disorders. Many nursing home residents suffer from dementia and do not realize that they need to eat or they may be uninterested in food altogether. These unavoidable physical causes as well as illness and adverse drug effects—including nausea, vomiting, diarrhea, sleepiness, and food interactions (that decrease the ability of the body to absorb vitamins and minerals), depression, swallowing disorders, mouth problems, and tremors—can and do affect the ability of residents to feed themselves. The choking incident described earlier demonstrates that it can actually render eating deadly.

Certified nursing assistants (CNAs) typically assist seven to nine residents with eating and drinking during the daytime, and as many as 12 to 15 residents during the evening meal. This contrasts with the ideal of one CNA for every two to three residents who require eating assistance. Staffing shortages contribute to malnutrition as well. Residents are fed quickly or forcefully or sometimes not fed at all.

Dehydration goes hand in hand with malnutrition. Two out of five nursing home residents suffer from some form of dehydration. Dehydration can result from diarrhea, the effects of medication, inability to perceive thirst, a physical inability to drink or swallow, or embarrassment related to incontinence. Most of the time, a resident's dehydration is due to inadequate care.

Pressure Sores

Pressure ulcers, also known as bed sores, pressure sores, or decubitus ulcers, are wounds caused by unrelieved pressure on the skin. When the body is left in the same position for too long, pressure prevents the flow of blood, which carries oxygen to the skin and tissues. Over time, the lack of oxygen causes the skin and tissues to die. Some experts believe that patients with poor diets may have a greater chance of developing bedsores or pressure sores.[102]

The sores usually develop over bony prominences, such as the elbow, heel, hip, shoulder, and back. Pressure sores are painful and dangerous, as patients who develop them are prone to life threatening infections. Not only are they a serious medical condition, they are also one of the important measures of the quality of clinical care in nursing homes. According to the 2004 National Nursing Home Survey, more than one in 10 nursing home residents (11 percent) had pressure ulcers, Stage 2 being the most common.

Federal regulations require facilities to ensure that:

- A resident who enters a facility without pressure sores does not develop pressure sores unless the individual's clinical condition demonstrates that they were unavoidable; and

- A resident with pressure sores receives necessary treatment and services to promote healing, prevent infection, and prevent new sores from developing.

Pressure ulcers are preventable. There is little room for deviation from this statement. The standard of care is for a bed bound patient to be turned and repositioned at least every two hours, especially if the resident is incontinent, because exposure to moisture from urine increases the risk of skin damage. Pressure ulcers are very often caused by an inexcusable failure to turn a patient frequently. These incidents are avoidable with appropriate staff to patient ratios. Nursing homes should provide an adequate number of qualified and properly trained staff so that they can detect early signs of pressure ulcers and follow up with treatment protocols.

Staffing Levels: What's Required and What's Reasonable?

If these were day care centers, we would collectively demand that there be enough qualified staff to watch the children's every move. So what staffing levels are required by law for caring for our aged constituents? Federal law requires Medicare- and Medicaid-certified nursing homes to have minimum staffing of a director of nursing (DON) who is a registered nurse (RN); an RN on duty at least eight hours a day, seven days a week; and a licensed nurse practitioner (LPN) or RN on duty the rest of the time. Studies have shown facilities with more RN staffing have, on average, a higher quality of care, but the average staffing levels of these facilities are far below the level recommended by experts, which is 0.75 RN hours per resident per day and 4.1 total hours of nurse staffing per resident per day.[103]

The Centers for Medicare and Medicaid Services report that facilities with staffing levels below 4.1 hours per resident day for long stay residents may provide care that results in harm and jeopardy to the residents.[104] Other studies also support a threshold level of 4.1 total nursing hours per resident day to ensure that the processes of nursing care are adequate. The optimum staffing level, according to the CMS, is one hour of licensed nurse time per resident and three hours of nursing assistant time per day. The data from a number of studies recently led the Institute of Medicine to recommend adding RNs 24 hours per day.[105]

Importantly, there are no federally mandated nurse to resident staffing ratios for RNs, LPNs, or nurses' aides (NAs), and there is no minimum level of staffing requirements for NAs, who provide most of the day-to-day care. There is only an unduly vague reference to "sufficiency." The fact that a facility of 50 residents has basically the same staffing requirements as a facility of 200 indicates the lack of specificity and adequacy of these federal requirements.[106]

All but 13 states have additional requirements above the federal ones; the others still rely on the irrationally vague federal standard. Fifteen states have higher RN standards, and 25 have higher licensed nursing standards. Eight states require an RN on duty 24 hours per day for facilities with 100 or more residents. Thirty-three states require minimum staffing for nursing assistants. The highest overall staffing requirement is in California, at 3.2 RN hours per resident day, excluding administrative nurses.[107]

There is ample evidence to support Mr. Evan's attorney's charge that these problems are especially rampant in for-profit nursing homes. They have lower staff ratios and higher deficiencies than non-profit and government facilities. A 2002 national study of nursing homes found that deficiencies in nursing home care were 40 percent higher in investor-owned facilities because of aggressive cost-cutting.[108] Thus, proprietary ownership and chains are associated with lower staffing levels and poorer process and outcome measures.[109]

This conclusion was again borne out by a study just last year. It was the first study to focus only on staffing and quality at the 10 largest national for-profit nursing home chains. It was led by Charlene Harrington—RN, Ph.D., and Professor Emeritus of sociology and nursing at the University of California, San Francisco (UCSF) School of Nursing—whose work is cited throughout this book. The chains were selected because of their success as defined in terms of growth and market share. They also wield a significant influence in the industry. These chains operate approximately 2,000 nursing homes and account for 13 percent of nursing home beds nationally.

According to Harrington, "Poor quality of care is endemic in many nursing homes, but we found that the most serious problems occur in the largest for-profit chains. The top 10 chains have a strategy of keeping labor costs low by decreasing staffing to increase profits. They are not making quality a priority."[110] The hard data showed that from 2003 to 2008, for-profit chains had fewer nurse staffing hours compared to non-profit and government nursing homes, even when controlling for other factors.

Collectively, total nursing hours in for-profit facilities were 30 percent lower than in government and non-profit nursing homes. Furthermore, the top nursing home chains were significantly below the national average for RN and total nurse staffing, as well as below the minimum nurse staffing advised by experts.

Are Profits and Good Care Mutually Exclusive?

Compared with the best nursing homes, the 10 largest for-profit chains were cited for 41 percent more serious deficiencies and 36 percent more deficiencies. Deficiencies include failure to prevent falls; infections; resident weight loss; pressure sores; poor sanitary conditions; resident mistreatment; and other issues that could considerably harm residents. Harrington's investigation revealed that the four largest for-profit chains had more deficiencies after being purchased by private-equity companies. I'm sure it will not surprise you to hear that these companies also had the sickest residents.

In the past I have heard from frustrated insiders that the nursing home industry is the most heavily regulated next to the nuclear energy industry. In fact, when I worked as an attorney for a nursing home corporation, my boss used to utter these words just before he got into his convertible Jaguar to drive to his boss' mega mansion. These complaints are typically followed by a statement about operating costs and low reimbursement rates and the concomitant lack of profits. Perhaps the clearest way to make my point is with a simple comparison. In 2008, the median annual salary of a certified nurse assistant—*the people who lay their hands on us and our loved ones*—was $23,193.[111] Let's contrast this with the $1 million salary that George V. Hager, Jr., the CEO of Genesis Healthcare Corporation, paid himself in 2006.[112] Despite my sincere acknowledgment that there's nothing wrong with trying to make a profit in the elder care industry, I still do not believe that there is any justification to pad a pocket to the detriment of a life.

I think it is obvious that I do not buy that there is no profit to be had in these facilities. Skilled nursing facilities have made enormous profits from Medicare. In March 2011, the Medicare Payment Advisory Commission (MedPAC), which advises Congress on Medicare policy, reported that Medicare payments increased faster than Medicare costs. In 2009, free-standing facilities had an average Medicare profit margin of 18 percent, an increase from 11 percent in 2003,[113] and one-quarter showed profit margins of nearly 25 percent.[114] In 2011, MedPAC reported that Medicare margins exceeded 10 percent for the ninth consecutive year.[115]

Logically, if these margins did not exist, why would they be traded by private-equity firms? According to the research firm Dealogic, since 2005 there have been at least 46 buy-outs of nursing-home operators worldwide. Private-equity firms now own three of the five largest chains of homes in the United States, including the biggest, HCR ManorCare, which was bought by Carlyle for more than $6 billion in 2007. These are the same firms that own the likes of Dunkin' Donuts. More important for the industry, according to the *Los Angeles Times*, toward the end of 2010 private equity firms had sold 246 companies for almost $90 billion, a 338 percent jump from 2009.[116] The evidence shows an increase in a host of problems with the advent of private equity capital in the nursing home industry.[117]

I consider myself an open-minded individual, but it remains my opinion that investors exaggerate the industry's precariousness. In short, there is no excuse for not paying for more staff. After all, why would General Electric purchase 185 facilities for $1.4 billion in 2006 if it was an unprofitable venture? It wouldn't. General Electric is the nation's largest industrial company, whose products range from jet engines to medical imaging machines. The gains from that deal were more than $500 million in just four years.[118]

The corporations purchasing these less-than-glamorous businesses are not full of bleeding-heart social workers. Nor do they have to be. But should they not strive to secure profits without sacrificing the lives of their clientele? Is a mission statement that involves providing an environment of care, comfort, and dignity for men and women in the twilight of life incompatible with making a nice living? Did they not see *Jerry McGuire*?! I would assume that they do quite of bit of forecasting and number crunching before committing to a $6 billion venture. Now if I could just un-grit my teeth, I will serve up the industry's excuse for providing substandard care *en masse*.

Where Are the Nurses?

So, with these profits, how can we believe that these facilities cannot afford to hire more staff? Let's start with blaming us pesky lawyers again. Can litigation costs and regulatory compliance issues justify proprietors' failure to ensure adequate staffing levels? I think not. In 2010, a nursing home class-action lawsuit in Northern California almost put the largest nursing home operator, Skilled Healthcare Group, Inc., out of business. In that case, the jury awarded more than $670 million to members of a class who alleged and proved that the facility did not meet minimum staffing levels.

Skilled Healthcare filed for bankruptcy protection in 2001. Nevertheless, the company, with its 14,000 employees, collected about $189 million in revenue and a profit of $8.9 million in the first quarter of last year, according to a filing with the Securities and Exchange Commission. Over the past five years it also acquired nursing homes in Texas, Illinois, New Mexico, Kansas, Nevada, and California. As part of the proposed settlement, Skilled Healthcare agreed to have an outside monitor track its nurse staffing levels for its 22 California locations for a two-year period. Skilled Healthcare shares *rose* 88 cents, or about 25 percent, to close at $4.38 one day after the settlement was announced. That's right. Investors made money from the misfortunes of the neglected.

Can the for-profit mega corporate facilities legitimately blame the Medicare and Medicaid reimbursement rates for any financial uncertainty they may face? State and federal governments pay about 70 percent of nursing home costs, and the government pays part or all of the costs for about 85 percent of all residents. Because the government pays such a large portion, nursing homes structure their care delivery system around the government payment system. Most will explain that the high Medicare reimbursement for rehabilitative services offsets the abysmal Medicaid reimbursement for long-term care and housing. Annual reimbursements from Medicaid are about $50,000 less per patient than from Medicare or private insurance, so Medicare funds help subsidize the 15 percent of a facility's population who are Medicaid patients.

Just as nursing homes are paid different rates for short-term vs. long-term patients, they are also paid different reimbursement rates for different types of post-acute care, depending on whether the patient's needs are simple or complex. Reimbursement is based on a relatively complicated formula. Many facilities assign residents to rehabilitation categories that give them the most favorable reimbursement rates, often without actually providing them with the number of minutes of therapy required in order to be placed in those categories.[119] But in doing so, they increase revenues and thereby increase profits.

Sadly and predictably, while reimbursements to facilities have increased, rehabilitation services for residents have actually decreased. The GAO reported that "The patients categorized into the two most common (high and medium) rehabilitation payment group categories typically received 30 minutes less therapy during their first week of care, a 22 percent decline."[120] Reimbursements for these billings were more than $4 billion above CMS expectations.

In October of 2011, in an effort to reduce the nation's huge federal deficit, Medicare cut its payment rates for nursing home residents by 11 percent, representing a $4 billion drop in annual payments. The intent was to better align Medicare payments with costs and to address billing manipulations by (mostly for-profit) facilities that garnered unwarranted reimbursements and resulted in the record profits set forth above. These facilities were finding loopholes in the reimbursement formula to game the system. The reduction affects what is known as "post-acute care" at skilled nursing facilities—services needed by seniors who have been hospitalized and who need to stabilize before returning to their own homes. CMS estimates that nursing homes receive about 20 percent of their total revenues for such post-acute care, meaning that their total revenues after these cuts would drop by a bit more than 2 percent.

CMS' reduction of overpayments to skilled nursing facilities is one effort to bring down health care costs and to ensure that payments are made to health care providers for services that are actually provided. These repeatedly documented overpayments have made skilled nursing facilities extremely profitable, but have not improved resident care as resident rehabilitation services have decreased.

Once Medicare reimbursements were cut, the industry claimed that it would have to cut staff. The stock prices of several publicly traded nursing home chains plunged immediately and the industry reacted with strong protests. However, this was a massive overreaction. Despite the overall reduction,

Medicare skilled nursing facility rates still remain high. In fact, the fiscal year 2012 reimbursement rates are 3.4 percent higher than 2010 rates.[121] It is difficult to muster sympathy for an industry whose hands got caught in the cookie jar.

What is more difficult to fathom is the audacity of the claim that cuts will erode the quality of care provided—as if the quality thus far has been a paragon of perfection. When facilities have been given <u>more</u> money by the government, it has *not* been used on patient care. Many government reports have documented that Medicare payments have been overly generous over the past 13 years. Just a few months ago, the Office of Inspector General (OIG) reported that Medicare payments to skilled nursing facilities increased by $2.1 billion (1.6 percent) between the last half of fiscal year 2010 and the first half of fiscal year 2011, even though beneficiaries' characteristics had not changed.[122]

In California, urged on by the pleas of the for-profit sector lobby, lawmakers passed the Nursing Home Quality Care Act of 2004. Prior to the new law, reimbursement from MediCal (what California calls its Medicaid program) was $124 per day. Afterward, nursing homes could be reimbursed $152 per day for the same type of care. With more money at their disposal, legislators assumed that nursing home operators would be able to employ more staff and therefore provide care to more medically fragile patients. That did not happen. Many nursing homes did not use their new income to increase staffing or their standards of care. Instead, they began to use their increased funding to fight claims of inadequate care. In short, they were able to bill taxpayers for the costs they incurred defending against lawsuits and challenging citations.

An investigation by California Watch found that 232 nursing homes either cut staffing after the increases, paid lower wages, or let caregiver levels slip below state-mandated minimum levels. California Watch also found that, of the 131 homes that reduced staffing, the median income was 35 percent higher than other homes that maintained staffing levels. Despite the funding increases, dozens of homes continued to operate below the state minimum standards and the numbers of complaints and statutory violations rose. Prior to the new enactment in 2004, there were 4,499 complaints against nursing homes. In 2008, there were 5,549—an 18 percent rise. Despite increased funding, the severity of injuries also became more pervasive.[123]

In the end, nursing homes are businesses, and one way many business owners increase profits is by cutting labor costs. Staffing accounts for more than two-thirds of a typical nursing facility's expenses, so employment cutbacks would be a likely place for expense reductions. But such cutbacks adversely affect the quality of care that seniors receive at such homes. According to a new survey by Avalere Health, nursing homes nationwide plan to lay off about 20,000 workers because of the Medicare cuts and plan to cancel a total of 400 expansion projects that could have created 20,000 new jobs.[124]

The CMS told *US News* that it does not "believe that nursing homes will respond to the payment changes by decreasing the quality of care furnished to patients." Some believe that while some shaky nursing homes will go under, stronger ones will be forced to choose residents carefully.[125] It is likely there will be a lot more screening of patients, resulting in rationed care. It is also likely that the problems outlined in this chapter will persist.

Should we allow some neglect because the alternative is self-neglect, for want of affordable housing and care for poorer old people? Is the threat of these for-profit businesses closing—removing a theoretically valuable housing option for our compromised citizens—a valid retort? Should this possible displacement raise our tolerance for these arguments from the private sector? Should we do an economic analysis much like Ford did with the Pinto?

These are heavy, complicated issues. More importantly, they are not abstract concepts, relevant only to some "other" person. If you are reading this book, they are relevant to **you**. Think about them, contemplate them, but above all else, use them to make good decisions about your future.

CHAPTER 6

Thanks Susan, Now I Am Just Freaking Out

I just dumped a big bucket of ice water onto your head, leaving you frozen, unable to move or think. You do not want to read on. But you must. You paid good money for this book. You did so because you wanted to learn. You have just arrived at the point of being ready to know what to look for if you need to go to a facility. There are some good ones out there, and I will tell you how to find them. So take back all of the negative thoughts you had about purchasing this material, and read on!

Searching for a nursing home is not easy, particularly considering the emotions involved and the limited time that is usually available. Unfortunately, there is no cookie-cutter formula to determine whether a particular facility suits your needs. Placement into a nursing home is usually not in one's playbook; it is a last resort when it's impossible to find the necessary care in any other setting. It is reactive rather than proactive. More often than not, the search is the result of a discharge from a hospital after an acute event such as a fall and resulting broken hip, a stroke, or some other acute incident.

Just yesterday, I was called by the wife of a man who was getting discharged from a hospital in three days. He has Alzheimer's, wanders, and is combative. The board and care home where he was residing could not care for him anymore and now, with less than 72 hours, his wife has to figure out what to do. She wants be able to see him all of the time, but she does not drive at night or on the freeway. These variables further limit her ability to make the best informed choice.

With the right preparation and information, she (and you) can find a place that works. This chapter is designed to provide you with detail about all of the things you should take into account as you conduct your search. To make things easier, I have provided you with a checklist that you can take with you as you visit facilities (see Appendix A).

Know Your Sources

Many people I help have relied on the Internet to find facilities for their parents or spouses, and with good reason—there is information online to be had. As with all information, though, you need to be informed about where it comes from and how it might be flawed. For example, in December of 2008, the Centers for Medicare and Medicaid Services (CMS) instituted a new Five-Star Quality Rating System for nursing homes nationwide to provide meaningful distinctions between high and low performing homes by reporting more than 19 different quality and safety measures. The ratings are available on the CMS Nursing Home Compare website (www.medicare.gov/nhcopare/), where facilities are assigned star ratings, from a low of one star to a high of five stars. Five stars purportedly indicate that a facility is "much above average" in its quality of care, and one star indicates a quality rating "much below average." The ratings are based on three factors: (1) health inspections; (2) staffing; and (3) quality measures.

The health inspections are carried out annually and conducted in accordance with current CMS inspection guidelines. Staffing information is based on the number of staff per patient, as reported by the nursing facilities themselves. Quality measure data are based on CMS' assessment of the prevalence of certain issues (such as bed sores and resident mobility) at the facility, relative to other facilities. Federal officials issue the top 10 percent of facilities in each category nationwide five stars, the bottom 20 percent one star and the middle 70 percent two, three or four stars, with an equal proportion (about 23 percent) in each category.

Importantly, the star system does not take into account penalties issued by state health departments. According to CMS, the federal government chose not to include state-level facility evaluations because the penalty criteria vary widely from state to state. This is problematic, however, because if a state inspector were to find a serious violation missed by a CMS evaluator, the Five-Star rating level would not be affected. Conversely, a strong compliance history with state regulations would not be reflected in the facility's rating.

This system has drawn quite a bit of criticism from groups ranging from legal analysts to senior advocates, as well as the nursing home industry itself. Patient advocacy groups worry that consumers may rely too heavily on what is potentially a somewhat faulty measure of quality. All question the system's accuracy and reliability as a tool for consumers who seek quality homes. Patients' rights groups have criticized the new rating system for its use of self-reported data. Two of the three sources of information used by CMS—facility staffing and quality measures—come from the nursing facilities themselves. These groups warn that nursing homes that are selective about the data they report could add to the unreliability of the ratings.

One criticism from the industry itself is that the system ignores the reality of caring for very old and frail adults. Inherent in our aging process is the degradation of bodies. We deteriorate. Pressure sores and other, often unavoidable complications of nursing home care such as urinary tract infections happen at a greater frequency once we reach a certain age. These facilities may provide great care to that segment of the population, yet may not be able to eradicate or prevent some conditions for which they receive deficiencies and low marks. This failure to account for different acuity levels between facilities can lead to very good facil-ities that provide services to a higher acuity patient base being judged poorly, and other facilities with lower acuity patients being rated higher than is deserved. Moreover, if this system persists, it may prove to be a disincentive for facilities to take high risk resi-dents, and an entire cohort may find itself homeless.

Even CMS has stated that the Five-Star system should be used as just one method of many to assess a nursing facility. It has indicated that simply because a facility is rated highly, it should not be assumed to be of top quality. Similarly, CMS has stated that nursing facilities that rate poorly in the Five-Star system are not necessarily poor-quality providers. I agree, and rarely counsel my families to rely solely on these measures when looking for a home.

So many times I have heard "I found this great site for…" But I would not put my blind faith in Internet sites or referral services that may be monetarily incentivized by a facility to place a resi-dent there even if the facility record is less than stellar. I know of referral companies whose salespeople wear badges that say that they are elder care consultants. When I asked one of them what her credentials were, she replied that up until a few years ago, she was in the entertainment industry. Another "elder care consultant" from that same company replied that she didn't finish college but that when she was in school, she was on track for a degree in social work. She was now in her late fifties. How can they look a family in the eye and tell them that they have the answers to their problems? Watch out. They are too often just salespeople for Internet sites. Likewise, a hospital discharge planner may offer valuable information about nursing homes, but her judgment may be impaired by the need to be expedient. These administrators are often overwhelmed. If the hospital needs to make room for another patient, any available bed at any facility may do. For these very reasons, I urge all of the families I work with to draw from as many sources as possible when selecting a nursing facility.

In fairness and for the sake of transparency, I do have facilities included as "Susan's Picks" on my website and I do get paid for the sponsorship. But I also engage in a tremendous amount of vetting before I agree to represent their interests. I spent the last three years researching everything I could about the long-term care industry. In short, if you do use an Internet site, find out who is operating it and what their research methodology is.

Choosing a Facility

Without a doubt, the most important indicator of how a facility will treat you or your family is a visit to the nursing home. This is far more important than the suggestion of a hospital administrator or the results of a potentially flawed rating system. It is imperative that you do groundwork. Do it before an acute incident. Do it now if you or your parents are old and there is a possibility that there will be a discharge from your local hospital into a facility at some point, because at that point there is very little time for careful thought and decision making.

In some cases you will visit a facility and know immediately that it's not for you. Other times you will need to do some investigating. In those cases, there are certain characteristics I want you to be on the lookout for, ranging from the physical location of the facility to the ways that it affects your senses. If you are a critical consumer, keeping all of these qualities in mind as you shop, you'll be more likely to find the place that's right for you.

Logistics

Although it seems as if I am stating the obvious, if you can manage to find a facility close to where you live or work, you will decrease the likelihood of neglect. There is no substitute for a pinch hitter, an alternate batter who can swing at a nurse or administrator if your needs are being ignored. Never underestimate the impact that frequent visits from friends or family will have on your mood or depression level. On balance, it might even be better to pick a facility that is more geographically desirable than another that has better ratings. As you will come to understand in Chapter 10, where I describe the importance of mental health, it is hard to quantify the impact of depression on chronic disease, but the correlation has been repeatedly noted.

Communication

We live in an ethnically and linguistically diverse culture with many individuals who have limited English proficiency (LEP). In recent years, a full 38 percent of applicants for Supplemental Security Income who were aged 65 or older asked to be interviewed in a language other than English.[126] In 2009, 57.1 million people (20 percent of the population five years and older) spoke a language other than English at home. These languages include Spanish, Portuguese, Russian, Hindi, Chinese, Vietnamese, Tagalog, and Arabic. According to a U.S Census study, the use of these languages is projected to increase, with Spanish projected to remain the most commonly spoken non-English language.[127]

Thankfully, there are a number of federal laws that address language access in health care settings. Virtually all health care providers must comply with Title VI of the Civil Rights Act of 1964, whose purpose is to ensure that federal money does not support activities that discriminate on the basis of race, color, or national origin. All 50 states have enacted laws concerning language access in health care settings. The National Health Law Program has published the state-by-state laws with citations to and a short description of each state's statutes and regulations regarding services to LEP persons in health care settings.[128]

You may or may not be among the group of Americans for whom English is not a first language. Regardless, when you are looking for a nursing home, you must pay attention to any issues that might prevent you from understanding the care you receive, or that could prevent your caretakers from understanding your needs and wishes. This is especially important if you have a hearing deficit or if you become cognitively impaired in any way, because in those cases communication will become even more difficult. If the facility does not have procedures and policies in place to facilitate clear lines of communication—whether because of language barriers or other factors—the obstacles could be frustrating at best, and dangerous at worst. This was a very real problem for one of my clients who had to rehabilitate in a facility after he fell and broke both shoulders; he asked that I include this in my book.

Philosophy of Care

It you are very lucky, you may stumble into a facility that has adopted the Eden Alternative or a similar philosophy of person-centered care. If you do, you will be much less likely to be treated like a commodity whose care results are quantitatively measured and bundled into a reimbursement case mix.

The Eden Alternative was created in 1991 by Dr. Bill Thomas and his wife Judy when he was a new medical director in a New York facility. They transformed the facility into a holistic environment housing older frail adults together with birds, cats, dogs, plants, a child care center, and a garden—all of which are cared for by the residents. Dr. Thomas' approach resulted in a decline in the need for restraints and drugs, and lower death rates and incidences of illness. Uncommunicative residents began to engage. Employee morale soared, producing an improved work ethic and fewer turnovers. At the moment, the Eden Alternative exists almost exclusively in private-pay only or nonprofit facilities because government funding does not reward the facility for the improvement of residents' health or for reductions in their medications—as you learned in the last chapter on corporate greed, government reimbursement is based on sicker residents receiving more care and lots of medications.

Recently, Dr. Thomas has extended his reform through the Green House Project, an approach to deinstitutionalizing care through newly constructed, communal living environments. This is just the type of radical approach to long-term care that I love. Nursing homes are torn down and replaced with small, home-like environments where people can live full and interactive lives. In 2005, the Robert Wood Johnson Foundation announced a five-year, $10 million grant to support the launch of Green House projects in all fifty states. To find out if your state is involved, go to the official Green House website at www.thegreenhouseproject.org. If you do not have this specific type of care available in your area, you can still look for facilities that have similar patient-centered qualities. If you can find one, you are more likely to be treated with honor and respect.

Physician Access

Good health care is not the exclusive province of the nursing home staff. You will need to ask if you can still see your personal doctors. Many doctors do not generally visit nursing homes or, at most, will only visit certain nursing homes. If you want to ensure that a certain doctor will visit a particular nursing home, check with the doctor as soon as possible. This implicates logistical issues again. It is important to be near your family and friends, but also your medical providers.

JCAHO Accreditation

Is the nursing home accredited by the Joint Commission on the Accreditation of Healthcare Organizations (JCAHO)? The Joint Commission is an independent, not-for-profit organization. It accredits and certifies more than 19,000 health care organizations and programs in the United States. The accreditation is recognized nationwide as a symbol of quality that reflects an organization's commitment to meeting certain performance standards. Most state governments have come to recognize Joint Commission accreditation as a condition of licensure and the receipt of Medicaid reimbursement.

Having accreditation may be positively associated with higher staffing levels and with higher quality of care. It means that the nursing home meets certain standards for care set by JCAHO. You can find information on the accreditation of nursing homes in your area on the web at www.jcaho.org. Select "Quality Check."

Special Care Units

The existence of dedicated special care units, such as those for persons with Alzheimer's disease, may also be associated with a higher quality of care thanks to the higher staffing levels that accompany them.[129] Some nursing homes advertise that they provide special care for dementia or other conditions, but these claims may simply be a marketing gimmick. In most states, there are no set laws or industry standards for specialization. If there truly is a specialized unit, ask the staff to substantiate the claim.

As a response to deceptive marketing practices and with the end goal of proper treatment for those who have Alzheimer's disease, the Alzheimer's Association created the document *Key Elements of Dementia Care*, a guide for providers (owners, operators, administrators, and hands-on staff) as they develop or enhance existing programs for people with dementia. This document defines, describes, and illustrates dementia-capable care in residential care settings such as retirement communities, board and care, and assisted living and skilled nursing facilities. Ask the facility if they know about this guide. You can look at it yourself before you check out a "special" unit and ask them:

Do they develop effective care/service plans? If they do, how? And how often are these plan revisited?

Do they individualize day-to-day care based on the resident's capabilities, physical health, behavioral status, and personal preferences? If so, how?

How can they ensure that the activities that make up a resident's daily experience reflect his or her preferred lifestyle while providing a sense of usefulness, pleasure, and success, and as normal a level of functioning as possible?

How are staff members trained? Do they understand the various components of Alzheimer's/dementia care? Do they have ongoing opportunities for education and support? How do staff members demonstrate dementia-capable skills and knowledge before caring for residents with dementia?

How does the environment (physical, social, and cultural) encourage and support independence while promoting safety?

Twenty-four leading organizations have expressed their support or acceptance of these recommendations. You can review the complete guide here: http://www.caassistedliving.org/web/pdf/resources/dementia_care_practice_recommendations.pdf.

Resident and Family Councils

Facilities with organized resident or family groups may have a higher quality of care.[130] The members of a resident organization—sometimes called a resident council—are usually residents of the home, and all residents have the choice to participate. While a resident in a nursing home has no fewer rights than anyone else, the combination of an institutional setting and the disability that put the person in the facility in the first place often results in a loss of dignity and the absence of proper care. These councils give control to many residents who feel like their lives have been taken over by their families and a heavily regulated system. Resident councils give members an opportunity to play an active role in their own lives and to influence decisions that affect them.

Likewise, family councils are usually organized and managed by the residents' families to improve the quality of care and life for the residents. They provide a vehicle for family members and friends to voice their concerns and request improvements for all residents.

Both types of councils ensure that facilities comply with the Resident's Bill of Rights. As discussed in Chapter 3, these rights came into existence in 1987 when Congress enacted the Nursing Home Reform Law, and the law has since been incorporated into the Medicare and Medicaid regulations. In its broadest terms, it requires that you, as a nursing home resident, be given whatever services are necessary to function at your highest possible level. Specifically, the law protects your right to:

- Be informed of your rights;
- Be informed, in writing, of the nursing home's policies;

- Be informed of the nursing home's services and charges;
- Be informed of charges not covered by Medicare or Medicaid;
- Be informed about your medical condition unless restricted by doctor's written orders;
- Participate in the planning of your care, including refusal of treatment;
- Choose your own physician;
- Manage your personal finances, or authorize someone else to manage them for you;
- Have privacy, dignity, and respect;
- Wear your own clothing;
- Use your own possessions while not infringing upon the rights and safety of others;
- Be free from mental and physical abuse;
- Be free from chemical and physical restraints unless authorized in writing by a physician;
- Voice opinions and grievances without fear of coercion and retaliation from others;
- Be discharged or transferred only for medical reasons;
- Appeal a discharge or transfer;
- Be accessible to visitors or to refuse visitors;
- Have immediate access by family members;
- Receive visitors during at least eight hours of a given day;
- Privacy and confidentiality for meetings or conversations with visitors; and
- Receive assistance from an advocate in asserting your rights and benefits.

Both the resident and family councils are governed by federal law. The Long-Term Care Ombudsman is mandated to protect resident and family rights in nursing homes and all other long-term care facilities. Any facility certified for Medicare and Medicaid must provide a meeting space, cooperate with the councils' activities, and respond to each group's concerns. Nursing facilities must appoint a staff advisor or liaison to the family council, and staff and administrators have access to council meetings only by invitation. While federal law specifically references "families" of residents, close friends of residents can and should be encouraged to play an active role in family councils, too.

When you are looking at different facilities, ask a nursing home staff member if you can get permission from the resident or family council's participants to attend a meeting so that you can hear what is at the heart of their concerns. Admittance may be a big hint about the climate of the facility, as will the attitude of the person you ask.

Payment

If you have relatively limited financial resources, you should confirm that the nursing homes you consider are certified to accept Medicaid reimbursement. Nursing homes certified to receive Medicaid reimbursement may not evict or transfer residents who, due to diminishing savings, become eligible for the Medicaid program after they have paid privately for nursing home care. However, many facilities will conduct pre-admission financial screenings to see how long your funds can sustain their fees. This is wrong, but they do it anyway.

Physical Restraints

Visit the facility often and at different unannounced times. When you visit during mealtimes, look to see if the residents are in the dining room and not in their rooms. Check to see if the food is the right temperature. Notice whether individuals who need help eating are attended to. How many people are being fed by one CNA? Are they eating canned green beans or does the food appear to be fresh? I recommend that any investigatory visit take place on the weekend or at night when many facilities maintain a skeleton staff (not literally, of course).

What you want to see during the day is that the residents are up and dressed, and engaging in activities. If the residents are restrained it could be a red flag that there are serious staffing problems. There are two types of restraints. One type, physical, is on the decline. The other, chemical, is on the rise. Physical restraints are defined as:

> Any manual method or physical or mechanical device, material or equipment attached or adjacent to the resident's body that the individual cannot remove easily, which restricts freedom of movement or normal access to one's body.[131]

Examples of physical restraints are soft bands used to secure wrists or ankles, roll belts (which secure the midsection), mittens to secure hands, vest restraints (which immobilize the upper body), and Swedish belts (to secure a patient in a wheelchair or Geri-chair, a reclining chair with a locking tray in front). These restraints are considered a form of medical treatment and, as such, can only be used under the direction of a doctor. But the doctor cannot simply order the use of a restraint. Rather, the medical reasons for the restraint must be spelled out, along with the circumstances under which and the length of time over which it can be used.

There are a host of dangers involved in the use of physical restraints, including but not limited to: falls, strangulation, loss of muscle tone, pressure sores, decreased mobility, agitation, reduced bone mass, stiffness, frustration, incontinence, and constipation. Aside from the health risks, it is obvious that the restraints are not compatible with dignity. Due to education and activism, the use of physical restraints on nursing home residents has been drastically reduced over the past 20 years. Medicare statistics verify that 21 percent of residents were restrained on a daily basis in 1991, compared to just 5.5 percent in 2007, the most recent full-year set of statistics available.[132]

Chemical Restraints

Although the use of physical restraints on residents in U.S. nursing homes dropped by more than half between 1999 and 2007,[133] the use of chemical restraints is on the rise. Recently there have been many reports of the sedation of older adults in these facilities.

Psychoactive drugs do have positive uses, including the treatment of depression. But many nursing homes routinely use psychoactive drugs as a substitute for needed care and as a form of chemical restraint. Drugs designed to treat schizophrenia and psychosis are instead used to drug residents with dementia into submission. These antipsychotic drugs are now viewed as extraordinarily dangerous for older people who do not need them. In April 2005, the Food and Drug Administration (FDA) issued "black box" warnings against prescribing atypical antipsychotic drugs for patients with dementia, cautioning that the drugs increased dementia patients' mortality,[134] nearly doubling the risk of death over three years.[135] In June 2008, the FDA extended the warning to all categories of antipsychotic drugs, conventional as well as atypical, and advised health care professionals, "Anti-psychotics are not indicated for the treatment of dementia–related psychosis."[136]

A recent issue of *Aging Today*, a publication by the American Society on Aging (of which I am a member), headlined: "Sedating our Elders: Beneficial Treatment or Mistreatment." That article, citing a 2010 University of South Florida study, revealed that within three months of admission, 70 percent of all residents are on at least one medication with psychoactive properties and 15 to 20 percent are on four or more. The majority of these individuals came with no long-term history of either psychiatric diagnosis or treatment.

The Centers for Medicare and Medicaid Services likewise reported that nationwide, between July and September of 2010, 39.4 percent of nursing home residents who had cognitive impairments and behavior problems but no diagnosis of psychosis or related conditions received antipsychotic drugs.[137] A smaller, but still significant, percentage of residents not at high risk (15.6 percent)—those without cognitive impairments or behavior problems—also received antipsychotic drugs.[138] Even more recently, the Office of Inspector General (OIG) for the Department of Health and Human Services released an unflattering report regarding the use and delivery of atypical antipsychotic drugs in our nation's nursing homes. Drawing from a random sample of records from a previous study of nursing home residents with Medicare claims for atypical antipsychotic drugs, the researchers determined that 99 percent of the records failed to meet federal requirements for the use of these drugs and one-third of the assessments were untimely or deficient. Only 9 percent of care plans were written with resident or family input, and only 3 percent were developed with a physician. These items are critical for effective resident care.[139]

Most experts agree that although there is mandatory nursing home staff training in mental health care in some states, there is little if any attention to such matters in state nursing home regulatory statutes. Studies have shown that education on non-psychopharmacological means of managing psychological problems is essential to remedying this problem.

On November 30, 2011, the Senate Special Committee on Aging held a special hearing titled "Overprescribed: The Human and Taxpayers' Costs of Antipsychotics in Nursing Homes." The hearing followed a May 2011 Inspector General's report that showed massive misuse of antipsychotic drugs to sedate and subdue residents with dementia. The Inspector General, along with other long-term care experts, testified at the hearing. All agreed that non-pharmacological options have been underused in dementia care and that they offer superior outcomes to antipsychotics.

Just last week I was called by a woman whose husband, 88, was transferred to a board and care home from the hospital after a surgery. Prior to surgery he had mild memory loss. Immediately thereafter, he suffered from what his physicians called sundowning syndrome. Although there is no established definition, sundowning is widely used to describe a group of behaviors occurring in some older patients with or without dementia at the time of nightfall or sunset. These behaviors include confusion, anxiety, agitation, or aggressiveness with increased motor activity like pacing, wandering, resistance to redirection, and increased verbal activity such as yelling.

His behaviors were too difficult for the board and care home to manage so he was shuffled to the nursing home where he was put on Risperidone, an antipsychotic drug used to treat the symptoms of schizophrenia. The black box warning on that medication states, "Studies have shown that older adults with dementia (a brain disorder that affects the ability to remember, think clearly, communicate, and perform daily activities and that may cause changes in mood and personality) who take antipsychotics (medications for mental illness) such as Risperidone have an increased risk of death during treatment. Older adults with dementia may also have a greater chance of having a stroke or mini-stroke during treatment."

Unfortunately, this is a fresh-off-the-press example of how medications are dispensed with reckless abandon and to families who place their trust in a mostly undeserving system. Hopefully my intervention will save this poor man's life.

Unfortunately, it is not easy to tell if residents are overmedicated. Just because someone is comatose does not mean that medication is the culprit. Someone in the last stage of Alzheimer's disease, for example, usually has difficulty eating and swallowing, needs assistance walking, and eventually is unable to walk, needs full-time help with personal care, is vulnerable to infections, especially pneumonia, and loses the ability to communicate with words. The important thing is that the staff is educated on these issues so that you can trust their care.

Deficiencies and Corrections

In addition to what you naturally observe by virtue of looking around, you have to affirmatively ask to see inspection records. Just because no deficiencies are listed for the most recent year, it does not mean that there have been no deficiencies—it may simply mean that the facility has yet to undergo its annual survey. As such, when you investigate a facility as a potential home, ask to see the most recent survey. This information, like the Five-Star system, should not be used as the sole measure of quality of care in a nursing home. While high numbers of violations generally indicate troubled facilities, a facility with low numbers may not necessarily offer excellent care. Conversely, an error rate of 6 percent on a measure should not be ignored, but if this error is just one or two percentage points over the allowable federal regulation error rate, the facility may not be fraught with problems.

Ask for previous reports. Nursing homes are not required to let you see the previous year's Form 2567 (shorthand for the Statement of Deficiencies and Plan of Correction), but if the administrator has retained them and gives you access to them, that is a good sign. By comparing several consecutive surveys, you may be able to see if there are any patterns of inferior care. Although I do not advise you to simply take the results of this or any evaluation at face value, the observations of the survey team will tell a far more detailed tale than any guided tour ever could. These reports cover approximately 180 individual health-related requirements and are laden with details of inspectors' observations, such as if food had been sitting out and was cold, or whether residents' diapers were soaked.

The facility's plans for correcting any problematic situations are also included on the 2567 form. By speaking with the administrator you can get a better idea of their plans of correction and their philosophy. If the administrator is too busy to help you understand the details or is annoyed by the inquiries, leave and do not look back. There may be valid explanations and the problems may have been addressed, but if the staff is not open to speaking with you about the reports, you have to wonder how open they would be to speaking with you if you had a problem yourself.

Remember, as anal and obsessive as inspection findings may seem, they most often don't go far enough. According to a 2008 Government Accountability Office report, state surveyors frequently miss or understate the extent of serious care problems. Between 2002 and 2007, federal surveyors did follow-up inspections of nursing homes that had recently been evaluated by their states. They found that 15 percent of the state surveyors had overlooked at least one problem carrying a risk of death or serious injury, such as untreated pressure sores or weight loss.[140]

Let's be frank. Finding a quality nursing home is like finding a good husband when you are on the brink of becoming an old maid. Just like it is hard to find a potential mate who brings no baggage to a relationship, it is hard to find a nursing home with no deficiencies whatsoever. In the case of a potential mate, you would just prefer that he come with a carry-on. Isolated events of infidelity as a youth could be forgiven if, through maturity, there have been solid and monogamous relationships. This would indicate an introspective and thoughtful human being. Likewise, in the case of a nursing home, you would prefer to see a rare transgression and signs of change for the better.

Isolated events in a facility that have been addressed through a well-thought-out plan of correction indicate a high level of responsiveness on the facility's part. A plan of correction sheds light on its ability and willingness to solve internal problems and provide good care for residents. If a nursing home has been cited repeatedly for the same or similar deficiencies in the past, its commitment to addressing and fixing the problems should be questioned. This is especially true if the facility files a similar plan of correction in response to the violation each time. If a facility is cited over and over for numerous or serious deficiencies, this may indicate real problems within the home.

Problems that present themselves repeatedly and problems that have the potential to become larger as time progresses are both indications of pervasive issues and you should turn around and wait for a better door to open.

Employ Your Ears

When you visit a facility, you want to hear people laughing and music playing. But there are also other things you should listen for, especially when you ask the right questions. You want to hear from other residents (and their visitors) that they are satisfied with the care they are receiving. If you are lucky, you will get an honest assessment from an employee. Not all of them toe the corporate line.

Make a point of talking to the administrator, director of nursing, and social services director and pin them down as to who at the facility bears the responsibility for certain tasks, and how the nursing home knows that those tasks are completed. It will be important for you to know how different therapies are performed and when. Ideally, therapists should be available throughout the day, seven days a week. You should ask the administrator and director of nursing for the therapists' qualifications and specializations, and find out whether or not they work exclusively for this nursing home. Obviously, for continuity purposes, it is better if the therapists are in-house.

Look at the activity schedule, and make sure that the activities are varied and plentiful. Ask the social services director if all activities are led by a member of the activities staff. If activities are the responsibility of the nursing staff or of volunteers, they are more likely to be canceled due to lack of time or preparation. You should also ask the social services director whether a resident council and family council meet regularly. Finally, you will want to know from the get-go who you can speak with or complain to if a problem arises. If you detect an attitude, turn around and walk out.

Use Your Brain

If it is not patently obvious by now, staffing levels are the biggest predictors of success in a facility. Compare staffing at different homes. Every facility that takes Medicare or Medicaid dollars must provide CMS with nurse staffing data, which is then converted into the amount of nursing time per resident. But the numbers should be used only as a rough guide, as they merely reflect the average number of nurses and nurse assistants in the two-week period before the most recent health inspection survey. Sometimes, administrators begin to beef up staff in anticipation of a survey; afterwards, they decrease the staff. Unaudited, staffing information accuracy must be taken with a grain of salt.

Also, many families hire nurses' aides to augment their family members' care. If it appears that there is a profusion of nursing staff, make sure that you are not misled. Find out how many of the caregivers are employed by the facility and how many are private duty professionals. If you tour a facility within two

months of its probable inspection and there seems to be an abundance of staff, try to come back a couple of months later.
Remember, this book is about planning, so you should be able to
engage this liberty. If not, you can always look at the Form 2567
and ask questions that arise from your review.

As important as the number of staff is the length of time they
have been with a facility. Unfortunately, specific turnover data for
particular facilities are not available, so this is the question I ask
within the first five minutes of any tour. If the housekeeping and
kitchen staff members have been there for years, you should give
the facility serious consideration. Annual turnover is especially
high among aides (50 or 100 percent annually), and they have the
most frequent direct contact with residents. If you find a facility
where a large number of these professionals have been there for
longer than a year, dig deeper—it may be a good place.

Just Follow Your Nose, Wherever It Goes

What you want to smell is what you smell in your own home:
nothing. Not urine. Not disinfectant. That lingering scent of Fabuloso might be an attempt to cover poorly monitored incontinence.
Every smell has a meaning, and none should be overlooked.

Be Sensible

We all know about the five senses listed by Aristotle: sight,
touch, hearing, smell, and taste, and I've talked already about how
you should use many of these as you seek a facility that suits
your needs. Although there is much debate in science circles as to
whether there are more, the five that we know of (and the sixth
that many of us agree exist) are all you really need to employ in
order to find a good home. Nothing can replace visiting a facility
and looking, feeling, listening, smelling and intuiting.

CHAPTER 7

There's No Place Like Home

By this point, it should be patently clear that you would not want to see your worst enemy in many of the nursing homes in this country. It is possible to find facilities that beat the odds, but it is not easy and, even in the best of circumstances, nursing facilities are not ideal. So, let's concentrate on how you can age in place. This chapter is devoted to those who want to stay at home.

AARP surveys consistently show that nearly 90 percent of people 65 and older want to stay in their homes as long as possible.[141] Three-quarters of Americans over the age of 45 believe that they will be able to stay in their current homes for the rest of their lives. These individuals respect the importance of planning for the future and believe that they are themselves planners. They also recognize the importance of key home features and commu- nity characteristics that can maximize comfort in later years. However, in reality, few have given a great deal of thought to the home or community characteristics they will need. And of those who have given it thought, only half believe that they will need to make changes to their homes as they age.[142] Again, this is why I am writing this book. We have to make our feet match our words and thoughts. We have to connect this disconnect with action.

Staying home does not necessarily mean that you will not be at risk for falling or becoming malnourished and dehydrated. Your physical environment must be evaluated, as must your ability to engage in activities of daily living (eating, bathing, dressing, toileting, ambulating) and your ability to maintain good health. Can you imagine waking up and sitting at the end of your bed thinking, as you stretch and yawn, "How will I get to the bathroom? And, once I am there, how will I get myself all the way down to the toilet and then back up again?" After that, you may wonder how you will get your shirt on or how you will make breakfast since you do not drive to the store anymore and there is no food. This is happening all across America and it is silently chipping away at the safety of our older adult population.

I have seen many older adults self-neglecting in their own homes, either because they are too stubborn and/or proud to allow help into their homes or because they have no one to organize assistance. Sometimes, there is cognitive impairment and a resulting inability to recognize that they are at grave risk of imminent harm to themselves.

I recently spoke to a fellow care manager who has been in this field for quite a long time, and she told me a story that I cannot get out of my mind. She worked for an organization that made house calls to isolated seniors. One day she was called by a landlord and asked to check on a woman living in one of his units who had dementia. When she and her volunteer opened the door, roaches streamed down and scattered. They were everywhere. The house was cluttered beyond imagination. The woman was removed and placed into a motel for a week while they fumigated—three times. The woman's hair had to be cut as it was matted and filled with roach nests and eggs. This is a true story.

Seniors may be afraid that asking for help is the first step in losing their independence. I will never forget meeting a woman who called me to come to her home. She was in her seventies and told me that she was afraid to put her garbage out because she thought her daughter-in-law was going to snatch her and throw her into a home. She was not paranoid. She was reacting to insensitive comments and ridiculous assumptions by her children. It was truly sad. It turns out that she was fine on all fronts. Her doctor, with whom I spoke, could not have agreed more. I was grateful to have provided this reality check.

When an older adult really wants to stay home, it is imperative that the environment is safe and that care will be delivered. I have two clients that illustrate this point.

Bill is a proud, tough, 85-year-old guy. He had a series of mini strokes (transient ischemic attacks) that gave rise to vascular dementia. One day I received a call from his son, a prominent and very busy professor. Bill was about to get discharged from a nursing home. He was a short stayer. He was hospitalized because he became extremely disoriented from failing to manage his medications. One day he took a triple dose of all seven of his medications and the next night he did it again. This led to dehydration and malnutrition. Not quite as serious but nevertheless devastating to his financial well being, in his stupor, he purchased a $50,000 parcel of property in some forsaken area of Nevada off of an infomercial. The doctor would not release William unless he went to another facility or unless he had demonstrable 24-hour assistance in the home.

Bill has what I like to call his Martin Crane chair from the series "Frasier." This is the 1960s recliner that Frasier Crane's father's bottom seemed glued to. Bill also loved his TV clicker. There was no way that he would be happy any other place than his home, but in order for him to stay there, he needed to hire a 24-hour caregiver. He did not have that kind of money, but luckily his home was paid off and he could get a reverse mortgage. (There will be a more thorough discussion of financing care, including reverse mortgages, in a later chapter.)

Now, let's take my client Winifred. As a retired teacher of thirty years, she just turned 80 and is sharp as a tack. She has lived in her apartment for 20 years. She has no children, no husband, and nobody else to call family. She still drives, but mostly during the day and on familiar routes, because she is limited by her eyesight. The only challenges she currently faces are her hearing and the fact that she is a fall risk. She is a very social person and is contemplating moving to an assisted living facility (explored in the next chapter) because she is a bit socially isolated. For now, however, she wants to stay put.

These two older adults represent two ends of the aging-in-place spectrum. Their needs range from not being able to manage a daily existence to only needing a modicum of assistance. In Bill's case, I had to evaluate his physical environment before he came home. Remember, any older adult could fall anywhere—one out of three adults age 65 and older falls each year. These data are probably quite conservative, as many of these falls go unreported for various reasons. Oftentimes my clients shrug a fall off as if it were a normal part of the aging process. Whatever the reasoning, the danger still exists for someone who has taken a fall, especially if they are elderly and alone. It is the job of the family or professional to reduce this risk. Bill's home was a bigger hazard than I could conjure for a good story. With jimmy-rigged wires all over the place, it really looked like the first throw on a pick-up sticks game. Even for a person without limitations, it was a mine field of tripping traps; for a man with a walker it was a disaster waiting to happen.

The grass in his backyard was as tall as my eight-year-old son. It covered pavers that Bill relied upon to get to his laundry line because he liked to air dry his belongings. Then there was the food in his refrigerator that was three months past its expiration date. Clearly, converting his home into a safe environment had its challenges, but with the help of a gardener and an electrician, we were ready to proceed with finding a caregiver. But exactly what level of service was needed? And, more importantly for you, what services were available?

In-Home Caregiving

You have many services available to you if you seek to age in place. It is important to understand the differences between home health care services and in-home care services. Examples of skilled home health care services include:
- Care for pressure sores or surgical wounds;
- Physical and occupational therapy;
- Speech-language therapy;
- Patient and caregiver education;
- Intravenous or nutrition therapy;
- Injections; and
- Monitoring serious illness and unstable health status.

Examples of in-home care services include:
- Help with basic daily activities like getting in and out of bed, dressing, bathing, eating, and using the bathroom; and
- Help with light housekeeping, laundry, shopping, and cooking.

Both of these models—which must be paid for privately or through long-term care insurance—can provide caregivers on part-time, full-time, overnight or 24-hour shifts. Live-in arrangements can also be made.

When an individual from an agency is hired (either for home health care or in-home care) the goal is to provide assistance with activities necessary to successful living. Most frail older adults need help with walking, bathing, and cooking. Even though it is often overlooked, almost all of my clients need assistance with medication management. Think about this: Have you ever been sick with the flu and taken your pain reliever and your cough medicine, and then looked at your antibiotic bottle and wondered if you already took that? Have you ever resorted to dumping the pills and counting them to see if you had already taken them? I have done this on countless occasions. Can you imagine what it is like for a mentally compromised person to keep track of 14 medications? Once I was called after my client's mother took seven doses of Aricept in two days and ended up in the hospital for an entire week. Home care—which can be arranged in a variety of ways, depending on your needs—is an essential part of avoiding these situations.

Home care offers other important advantages. For example, we cannot overlook the impact that social isolation can have on an older adult. Many of my clients have simply stopped eating because they had no one to cook for them and no one to eat with, and losing too much weight left them susceptible to chronic illness. And another benefit of using an in-home care agency that is typically overlooked is the respite it can provide to someone who has chosen the laudable but very difficult path of family caregiving.

When I assist a family in hiring a caregiver, I make sure that the individual has gone through numerous background checks including a DMV check, a drug test, and a criminal background check. If I am working with an in-home care agency, I make sure that these checks are part of their hiring protocol. It goes without saying that it is imperative that the older adult—whether that is you, or your loved one—be part of the process. Sometimes, my clients interview five or more caregivers. If the agency has a problem with that, move on.

In-home care companies usually charge between $16 and $27 an hour. The fees for someone to stay 24 hours a day, seven days a week are typically between $200 and $275 a day or between $6,000 and $8,000 a month. If you need two 12-hour shifts because you or your loved one wakes up and wanders, is a fall risk, or engages in potentially dangerous activities such as turning on the stove, etc., it will be considerably more expensive. If you're eligible for Medicaid, some personal care services in your home may be covered. However, individual states do not do a great job of vetting the caregivers that they send to people's homes, so you must be especially vigilant.

In this economy, there are many people looking for jobs and it is very tempting to use an Internet site to find a caregiver who will only charge you $10 an hour, but this can often be very dangerous. According to a California Senate report, lax oversight of in-home care agencies is opening the door for caregivers with criminal backgrounds to offer services to the elderly and disabled. A California Senate Office of Oversight and Outcomes review of advertisements on the site craigslist.org for in-home caregivers uncovered five confirmed cases where the individuals offering services had extensive criminal records, including arrests for burglary, narcotics trafficking and prostitution. It also found that more than 25 percent of caregivers identified in media reports as being convicted or accused of wrongdoing on the job had previous offenses on their records.[143] Most states regulate private in-home caregivers; for a list of which states license and certify these companies, please see Appendix B.

There can be and often are nonfinancial costs associated with picking a caregiver. Obviously the biggest potential cost is elder abuse. Without criminal background checks, you may unwittingly open your home and finances to someone who has shown a willingness to exploit or harm others. What is the price point on you or your parent getting verbally or physically assaulted? Is it the difference between $10 and $15? Would you pay an additional $5 an hour to ensure that you or your loved ones are truly safe?

There is also the business side to hiring your own caregiver. When you choose to go that route, you may become an employer. To mitigate these unforeseen costs you must understand the rules associated with hiring your own personnel. If a caregiver performs household services in or around your home, and what is to be done and how it is done are subject to your will and control, that caregiver is your "household employee." It does not matter whether you exercise this control, as long as you have the legal right to control both the method and the result of the services. The two usual characteristics of an employer-employee relationship are:

      1) The employer can fire the employee.
      2) The employer gives the employee tools and a
         place to work.

To see if you are considered the "employer" of a "household employee," check IRS Publication 926, The Household Employer's Tax Guide for details. If an employment relationship is established, you may be responsible for employment taxes and unemployment insurance. You will also be required to withhold and pay Social Security and Medicare taxes on those employees paid $50 or more in cash wages during a calendar quarter. Also, pursuant to the Federal Unemployment Tax Act (FUTA), employers are required to make quarterly tax payments on domestic wages of $1,000 or more during a calendar quarter for the current or previous year. States also have unemployment tax requirements. And you must not forget to give your household employee copies B, C and 2 of IRS Form W-2 (Wage and Tax Statement) by January 31 after the year in which wages were paid.

As an employer, you are responsible for verifying that your employee is eligible for employment in the United States. Your local office of the Immigration and Naturalization Service will supply you with Form I-9. This form lists the documents that every worker must show to an employer to verify work eligibility in this country. You are required to keep this form and photocopies of the supporting documents in your files for at least three years after the date of hire.

And finally, what happens when that caregiver injures her back on the job? If you do not have a worker's compensation rider on your insurance policy, you will be footing the bill for her injury. There are laws holding employers liable for on-the-job injuries to household employees. Do not assume that your home-owner's insurance will cover injuries sustained by your privately hired caregiver. In fact, many times your policy will specifically NOT COVER injuries sustained by household employees.

Even if you have an in-home care company working in your own or your parents' home full time, and even if it is with a great company, they cannot be left to their own devices. You have to micromanage their work. If you can't, then you have to have a geriatric care manager do that for you. Here's why:

I had a man call me from Denver to check in on his father in Los Angeles who had three—count them, three—caregivers on three different shifts. He was on 14 medications, was afraid to get up and walk from his chair (and consequently often missed doctors' appointments), and was incontinent. His wife of 40 years told him she was leaving him one day in the hospital after he awoke from emergency open heart surgery.

In our conversation he told me that his father's caregivers did not sleep over. They got there at 9:00 a.m. and left at 8:00 p.m. Every day, he woke up at 5:00 in the morning and would just lie in bed waiting for someone to help him. That is four hours, after sleeping for nine hours. Had these caregivers ever heard of bed sores? Did they know how easily an older adult's skin could break down, especially if he is incontinent and marinating in a urine-soaked diaper? Upon receiving my report, the son had a ramp installed so that his dad could get into the car for the doctor and he hired an agency instead of the hodgepodge of casual CNAs that he had put in place after an Internet search for caregivers. Since he was not available to manage the caregivers, I also suggested he hire me or put his father in a board and care, but he did not proceed with these recommendations.

Why would a caregiver from an agency need to be managed by you or a geriatric care manager? First, caregivers do not get paid a lot of money. The company may charge $18–$25 an hour, but the employee gets paid $10–$12 per hour. Although usually caring and lovely, these workers typically do not speak English very well and are not well educated. Sometimes, this means they need social schedules and menus created. I have seen some otherwise great caregivers purchase Lean Cuisines or other frozen food for clients and just let them sit and watch television instead of planning nutritious meals and finding engaging community activities to take them to. If you or someone else does not watch over the older adult, preventative care can get lost. I often schedule doctor, dentist, and eye care appointments for my clients and then direct the caregiver to take them. Just yesterday, I called a local library to organize an opportunity for one of my clients to read to toddlers two times a month. She has already gone to a senior writing group that I organized, and her mood is considerably less dark.

A geriatric care/case manager, such as myself, is a professional who assists individuals and their families in remaining in their own environments, healthy and independent, as long as possible. The care/case manager is trained and experienced in assessment, coordination, monitoring and direct delivery of services. As a professional, the person should have a clinical or graduate degree in social work, psychology, or one of many health care fields, including, but not limited to, nursing, occupational therapy, and physical therapy. Fees may range from $60 to $250 per hour. Since geriatric care/case managers are not licensed or overseen by any regulatory agency, make sure you know the qualifications of the person you hire to perform this function. You can find a geriatric care manager through the National Association of Professional Geriatric Care Managers (www.caremanager.org) or by word of mouth in your community.

Technology and Other Accommodations

Now let's switch to my client Winnie, who does not need in-home care or any of the services thus far explored. She has hearing deficits, and talking to her on the telephone is like being in a Laurel and Hardy routine. But, jokes aside, not being able to communicate on the phone can have serious consequences. It can cause irritability, embarrassment, tension, stress, anxiety, depression, and negativism. Worse, it can lead to avoidance of social activities and withdrawal from personal relationships and loneliness. Most importantly it can endanger personal safety and general health.

For example, what if the pharmacist calls and changes a dose of medication, or the doctor's office calls with an appointment or test results and a hearing challenged older adult feigns hearing by saying "Yes, okay." A lot of people who have difficulty hearing a conversation will do this—they fake their way through it. What if there is an emergency and the front line worker is trying to assist only to repeatedly be met with "What did you say?"

Luckily, there is a lot of new technology that can ensure that you can stay independent in your home as long as possible. Technology need not be complicated. One of the most important hearing-related products is a smoke alarm with amplified sound. And while we often associate technology with electronics, it can also be surprisingly simple. Grab bars or a frying pan, as well as a calculator or a notebook fall into this category.

For Winnie, I recommended a CapTel captioned phone. It is similar in concept to captioned television, where spoken words appear as written text for viewers to read. The phone looks and works like any traditional phone, with callers talking and listening to each other, but with one very significant difference: word-for-word captions are displayed on the phone's built-in screen so the user can read the words while listening to the voice of the other party. If Winnie has difficulty hearing what the caller says, she can read the captions for clarification. It saves conversations so that she can go back and review them later. This has proved invaluable to her.

The specific items that exist to assist people are too innumerable to list here. For example, ambulation devices run the gambit from grab bars and walkers to lifts that can help a person get up the stairs to the bedroom or bathroom. My all-time favorite client had a stair lift installed. When I came to visit her she had to demonstrate it to me. She was tiny. She would get onto the lift at the bottom of the stairs and ride it straight up and down like a rollercoaster at Six Flags, all the time squealing "wheeee!" Aside from the entertainment value, this simple tool enabled her to stay in her home. Another client had a special lift made for his home because his stairs zig zagged up. Without this, he would have had to go into a board and care facility.

Being able to walk into a bathtub can help an older adult achieve a highly desired sense of independence. This is especially so for those who have previously been dependent on someone else for every need. A walk-in tub enables the user to safely undress, bathe, and dress again without full dependence on a nurse or assistant. This equipment is yet another example of products that can be utilized to enable you to age in place.

In a later chapter I will describe all of the laws that you must be familiar with. At this point, it is important that you know that, pursuant to the Americans With Disabilities Act (ADA), landlords must allow disabled tenants to make reasonable modifications to their living units or common areas at their own expense, if they are necessary for the person to live comfortably and safely in the unit.[144] In other words, you have the right to modify your living space to make it safe and comfortable. Examples of modifications that might be undertaken include:

- Lowering countertops for a tenant who uses a wheelchair;
- Installing special faucets or door handles for someone with limited hand use;
- Modifying kitchen appliances to accommodate a blind tenant; and
- Installing a ramp to allow wheelchair access to a raised living room.

There are stipulations, however. The modifications must be reasonable and made with the landlord's prior approval. Moreover, the landlord is entitled to ask for a description of the proposed modifications, proof that they will be done in a workman-like manner, and evidence that you are obtaining any necessary building permits. Additionally, if you propose to modify the unit in a way that will require restoration when you leave (such as the re-positioning of kitchen counters), the landlord may require you to pay into an interest-bearing escrow account the amount estimated for the restoration. (The interest will belong to you.)

If you are a disabled veteran or service member, please also know that the VA has three main grant programs to assist with necessary home modifications. Two of these are the Specially Adapted Housing (SAH) grant and the Special Home Adaptation (SHA) grant. These are designed to help provide a barrier-free living environment that affords you a level of independence you might not otherwise enjoy, such as creating a wheelchair accessible home if you have specific service-connected disabilities. The grants range from $12,000 to $62,000. Much smaller grants for non-service related disabilities are also available under Home Improvements and Structural Alterations (HISA). For more information about these VA grants, call 800-827-1000 or go to the VA website (http://www.benefits.va.gov/homeloans/).

Of course, you have probably heard about emergency alert devices that can assist you if you fall. Most companies offer portable versions so that if you are gardening or doing laundry away from a central system, you can push a button on a necklace, watch, or wristband and be contacted on the telephone and/or an intercom. According to the CDC, over 19,700 older adults died in 2008 from unintentional fall injuries.[145] My husband's aunt once fell and lay on the floor for seven hours until my mother-in-law happened to stop by. This could have proved fatal. If she had this device, she would have been helped immediately.

And with the push toward virtualization in almost every capacity, it was only a matter of time until doctor visits for checkups went virtual, as well. There are now web-based programs that allow seniors to connect to their doctors via web cam for face-to-face medical consultations. Service charges run from $40 to $50 per "visit." There are also mobile physicians who make good old-fashioned home visits just like Marcus Welby, M.D. It is unclear, however, whether insurance companies will view this as an actual visit that is covered under medical plans.

Have a Plan!

Finally, I would be remiss in my self-imposed duties if I did not mention the importance of making sure that you have a disaster plan. Whether you scoff at global warming or attribute the seemingly more omnipresent severe weather events to that phenomenon, in the end, when the walls come tumbling down, we all have to be prepared. Why is a disaster plan especially important for older adults? Shall I remind you of what happened in New Orleans?

According to Grantmakers in Aging, which has been active in the hurricane relief effort, people aged 60 and older comprised 15 percent of the area's population prior to Hurricane Katrina. More than 70 percent of those who died in Louisiana as a result of the hurricane were elderly; many of the 200 people who died as a result of the hurricane in Mississippi were older adults. More alarming, data from the Louisiana Department of Health show that almost 70 nursing home residents died in their facilities. Many were allegedly abandoned by their caretakers.

Imagine an older adult with a chronic illness, such as diabetes or breathing disorders, who might suffer in a disaster because she is unable to take her medications or lacks access to the technologies that help her function independently. A detailed, manageable plan could help guide her (and you!) through a crisis. If you would like a great example of such a plan, the Red Cross has a 32-page guide entitled Disaster Preparedness for Seniors by Seniors. You can call the Red Cross at 1-800-RED-CROSS to find out how to get your own copy.

A Special Note for Caregivers

If you are reading this book as an adult child of someone who is committed to aging in place, you should know that there exist various technologies that can help you stay connected to your loved one. Devices currently being tested enable long-distance caregiving. There are in-home systems such as sensors and devices that passively monitor whether a person is up and moving around. For example, kitchen use can be monitored with both motion sensors and micro door sensors (small open/close detection sensors) mounted on the refrigerator, silverware drawer, or on a commonly used food cupboard or pantry. The data transmission uses a two-way modem in the security panel, which pages all events to a central location. This can help monitor eating habits, so that you will know if your loved one is really getting nourishment, and more specifically, which foods are being consumed. Sensors placed on doors work well if someone with Alzheimer's tries to wander from the home.

As an adult child concerned about your mother living alone, imagine checking her house from your work desk to find that a companion robot has given her medicine and helped her out of bed and into a chair. This is the vision of the future offered by Bill Gates who, in a recent issue of *Scientific American*, argued that the robotics industry is on the cusp of a big expansion. Currently, the Carebot is a prototype robot that's still being tested as an aide to nurses in homes and—in the not too distant future—hospitals. It can sense movement and will follow a person around a home. It offers a video surveillance system so that family members or professional caretakers can keep an eye on parents or patients and, if there's no response from the senior, it can contact you by phone to alert you that there might be an issue.

Have you ever heard of an accessory dwelling unit (ADU)? Me neither! Until I started doing this research, I did not know that I could add this to my single-family home. These have also been called "in-law apartments," "accessory apartments," or "second units." (As a parent, I am already thinking of another name: "Get this kid out of my house dwelling.") It is a second living space within a home or on a lot, with a separate living and sleeping area, a place to cook, and a bathroom. Space such as an upper floor, basement, attic, or space over a garage may be turned into an ADU.

Of course, this option is contingent on a pass from your local zoning office. The cost is dependent upon how big a space is dedicated and the local costs for building materials and workers. With the average base rate of assisted living at $3,500, it is conceivable that you will break even on the construction of a 900-square-foot dwelling within six months. After that, the only expenses would be future costs of in-home assistance. If you can live with your mother-in-law, this may work for you. But you know what they say… Behind every successful man stands a devoted wife and a surprised mother-in-law.

One could argue that all of these devices and services may simply isolate seniors. I tend to agree. Anytime a senior is left alone, this is a risk. That is why it is imperative to seek out adult day care centers, adult day health care centers, and senior centers in your area.

Adult Day Care

Adult day care centers are designed for older adults who can no longer manage independently, or who are isolated and lonely. They offer a planned program of activities designed to promote well-being through social and health-related services. Nutritious meals that accommodate special diets are typically included, along with afternoon snacks. A well-run adult day care center can benefit both the senior and the caregiver. Participants can benefit from socializing with others and receiving needed care services. Caregivers can benefit from the break in caregiving duties while knowing that a loved one is in good hands.

According to the National Adult Day Services Association (NADSA), there are currently more than 4,600 adult day care centers nationwide. Each state provides different regulations for the operation of adult day care centers, although NADSA offers some overall guidelines in its Standards and Guidelines for Adult Day Care, including a minimum staff to participant ratio of one to six. This ratio can be even smaller, depending upon the level of participant impairment. If a program serves a large proportion of participants with dementia, for example, the ratio of staff to participants should be closer to one to four.

Good candidates for adult day care centers are seniors who:

- Can benefit from the friendship and functional assistance a day care center offers;
- May be physically or cognitively challenged but do not require 24-hour supervision;
- Are in the early stages of Alzheimer's disease;
- Are mobile, with the possible assistance of a cane, walker or wheelchair; and
- Are continent (in most cases).

When you contact an adult day care center you've chosen to consider, ask the following questions:

- Who owns or sponsors the adult day care center?
- How long has it been operating?
- Is it licensed or certified (if required in your state)?
- What are the days and hours of operation?
- Is transportation to and from the adult day care center provided?
- Which conditions are accepted (e.g., memory loss, limited mobility, incontinence)?
- What are the staff's credentials, and what is the ratio of staff to participants?
- What activities are offered? Is there a variety of individual and group programs?
- Are meals and snacks included? Are special diets accommodated?

Of course, you should always visit the center to see if it is a good fit. Be sure to bring a site visit checklist with you each time. The National Adult Day Services Association offers the following suggestions:

- Did you feel welcome?
- Were the center services and activities properly explained?
- Were you given information regarding staffing, programming, and costs?
- Is the facility clean, pleasant, and free of odor?
- Are the building and site wheelchair accessible?
- Is the furniture sturdy and comfortable?
- Are there loungers and chairs with arms for relaxation?
- Is there a quiet place in the center?
- Did the staff and participants seem cheerful and comfortable?
- Are participants involved in planning activities?

Adult Day Health Care

A social adult day care center, which I just described, is different from adult day health care, which usually requires a health assessment by a physician before an individual is admitted into the program. These centers typically use the term "Adult Day Health Care" (ADHC) in their names, often provide physical, occupational, and speech therapy, and are usually staffed with an RN and other health professionals. A third, related type of day care provides social and health services specifically for seniors with Alzheimer's or related types of dementia. Adult day health care centers provide health monitoring, social contact, meals, and activities for older people who are not thriving at home. The participants return to familiar surroundings at the end of the day.

The existence of these facilities is in great peril because of their heavy reliance on Medicaid dollars, which are being cut as we go about our days. There are currently several states that are still struggling with significant budget deficits and, as a result, some have decided to cut funding for adult day care services. The

American Recovery and Reinvestment Act of 2009 increased federal Medicaid funds for states suffering a decline in tax revenues and an increased demand for Medicaid funding, but this additional funding is set to expire at the end of 2012. However, there is support for a six-month extension to keep funding at current levels. Regardless, expiration of the American Recovery and Reinvestment Act could dramatically impact adult day care providers, the elderly, and their family caregivers.

Senior Centers

The most common objection I encounter when I recommend a local senior center is that they are "for old people." Much to my surprise, these words roll from the tongues of octogenarians. And yet, even baby boomers who are approaching retirement can benefit from the new programs and opportunities that are always being developed to meet the needs and interests of this dynamic generation of older adults. According to the National Council on Aging, research shows that older adults who participate in senior center programs experience measurable improvements in their physical, social, spiritual, emotional, mental, and economic well-being.

Senior centers provide a wide range of services and activities such as educational opportunities, counseling and support groups, volunteer opportunities, and wellness programs. Almost all senior centers have an activities director and a social worker available to assist clients with referrals to professionals. Some centers offer meals, help with financial and medical paperwork, transportation to and from the center, and shopping trips and outings. They also open the doors to friendships between seniors.

Many senior centers provide some congregate meals—perhaps a breakfast or lunch for a group of seniors—for little or no cost. All seniors 60 years of age and over, regardless of income, are eligible to participate in and receive free meals in a congregate meal setting. For little or no cost to seniors, these programs contribute greatly to nutrition and health while providing an important opportunity for socialization and friendship.

If you cannot get to a senior center, you can still avail yourself of meal delivery programs. These programs are not designed to take the place of every meal, but are offered for the convenience of you and your family. Availability depends upon the financial and volunteer resources of the local agency. Only those with a need will be considered, and this need may have to be verified.

Meals-on-Wheels is a term that most people are familiar with and in fact it has become more of a descriptive term than a name. Many programs call themselves Meals-on-Wheels for the sake of understanding and recognition. Programs using the name almost always deliver meals to your home, though some also have congregate meal service arms as well. If you are only *temporarily* disabled such as after an accident, injury, or surgery, there may be a limited amount of time that you can be in the program. Once recovered and able to shop and cook for yourself again, your services would probably be terminated to make room for someone else.

There is a cost associated with these programs, but often it is simply a suggested donation. Some programs base these amounts on income level or some other criteria. Many programs supply meals on a sliding cost scale where those with higher income pay a higher percentage of the cost of their meals. Hardship cases sometimes get preferential prices or no-cost meals. An average cost or suggested donation would be some-where between $2 and $5 per meal—but again, this varies. To determine what costs may apply, you should contact your local program office. You can contact the Meals on Wheels Association of America at 703-548-5558 or through their website (www.mowaa.org).

Grassroots and Innovative Alternatives

There are some grassroots efforts going on across the country that cater to individuals who are unwilling to be ushered by developers into cookie-cutter senior housing and told what to do and when to do it by people like me—a social worker-type half their age. One example of this is the Beacon Hill Village, started in 1999 by a group of friends who wanted to stay engaged in their own neighborhood in the vibrant city of Boston. They recognized that they might need support in the future and, looking beyond conventional solutions that allowed self-directed care, they created a self-supporting non-profit 501(c) (3) organization. It is funded by membership fees of $500 to $700 a year and donations.

The Beacon Hill Village model is a concierge-like service that seniors can call for anything they need, including handyman services, transportation, shopping, and health care. These services are usually supplied at negotiated discount prices. The Village also supplies all sorts of social activities and outings, thus keeping seniors active and ending isolation.

In 2006, Beacon Hill published *The Village Concept: A Founder's Manual* to share some of its experience in a hands-on, tell-all style that many groups have found very useful. The document is intended to guide others through the complexity of creating a business plan and surveying community needs. It encourages imitations and describes mistakes as well as successes. The manual is priced at $300 for nonprofits and neighborhood groups and $500 for for-profits and municipalities.

Some cite the fact that the Beacon Hill Village and others like it are mostly found in densely populated, relatively affluent urban or suburban communities as an impediment to mass implementation. Moreover, the members are overwhelmingly white—more than 90 percent, according to a survey last year by the University of California, Berkeley—suggesting that the village movement is best described as a boutique phenomenon.[146] However, many villages have subsidized memberships for those who cannot afford the full price. About one-quarter of Beacon Hill's members are in the subsidized program, and there is a small waiting list for inclusion.

Another innovative program is the Program of All-Inclusive Care for the Elderly (PACE). PACE offers an opportunity for individuals without the financial resources to pay privately for programs to upgrade their living quarters or to pay a fee to belong to a cooperative. The program provides comprehensive long-term services and supports to Medicaid and Medicare enrollees. (These people are euphemistically called dual eligibles.) PACE provides community-based care and services to people if they meet certain conditions. They must:

- Be age 55 or older;
- Live in the service area of a PACE organization;
- Be state-certified as eligible for nursing home care; and
- Be able to live safely in the community.

Through PACE, an interdisciplinary team of health professionals provides individuals with coordinated care. For most participants, the comprehensive service package enables them to receive care at home rather than in nursing homes. It provides coverage for prescription drugs, doctor visits, transportation, home care, hospital visits, and (whenever necessary) nursing home stays. Many PACE participants get most of their care from staff employed by the PACE organization in the PACE center. PACE centers meet state and federal safety requirements and include adult day programs, medical clinics, activities, and occupational and physical therapy facilities.

Even if you live in assisted living facility, you can still participate in PACE. While PACE will not cover the costs of room and board, it *will* pay for medical costs. It is a good option if you don't want to move to a nursing home but need additional care and have high medical bills. Unlike nursing homes, assisted living facilities do not accept Medicaid, but PACE can help ease the financial burden of residing in one by absorbing your medical costs.

PACE programs provide a model for reducing unnecessary hospitalizations and rehospitalization through effective care management. One study found that PACE enrollees spent fewer days in the hospital than comparison subjects. The researchers concluded that the savings of reduced hospital use could offset the costs of an expanded set of services, all the while maintaining quality.[147] The implications for long-term care policy and service delivery seem obvious.

One word of warning: PACE providers are paid by Medicaid like a managed care plan in which a set amount is paid per person, whether services are used or not. Thus, there can be a substantial estate recovery claim after a Medicaid beneficiary dies.

Currently, 76 PACE organizations operate in 29 states. Historically the program only existed in urban neighborhoods, but PACE has recently made inroads into rural America. The Rural PACE Pilot Grant Program, established under the Deficit Reduction Act of 2005, gave fifteen providers start-up funds to develop PACE organizations serving rural elders with limited access to quality health care services. Rural elders are more likely to be poor, have less formal education and be in poorer health.[148] Rural areas also have a higher proportion of people ages 65 and older and have higher nursing home utilization. Rural PACE programs provide an alternative to nursing homes for these older frail adults.

For a list of PACE organizations nationwide, visit its website (www.cms.hhs.gov/pace/pacesite.asp). For information about community services, call your local area Agency on Aging, Aging and Disability Resource Center, or Center for Independent Living.

I hope that from this chapter you were able to breathe a sigh of relief about your own independence or that of a loved one. The ability to age in place takes coordination of many products and services, which, as logic dictates, increase in intensity as time marches on. Nevertheless, it is an accomplishable goal. Of course, it requires the financial wherewithal to do so. How to finance all types of care for all people—even those who have moderate to little income and assets—will be explored later, in Chapter 11. For now, let's turn to a discussion of some of the other alternatives to nursing homes.

CHAPTER 8

There's No Place Like Home That Is Not Your "Home"

I am not a materialistic person. Sure, I have a strong aesthetic sense, but I don't need inanimate objects to make me happy or to maintain a state of happiness. For me, home is a place to keep my family warm at night and to entertain. My pets think of it as a watering hole and a place to empty their bladder, but that is a whole other story. My point is that because I see it as four walls that serve a function, I can detach from it. If it does not serve me anymore, when the 17 stairs leading up to my kitchen and bedroom are too difficult to climb, I will move. Period.

You know by now that this book is designed to keep you out of a nursing home, but there is a lot of confusion about the other long-term care options that exist. Often when I speak to seniors about leaving their homes, they think that means being institutionalized in a nursing home. They do not know that they could be living in a hotel-like environment with care-free days devoted to fun, friends, great food, and NO HOUSE-KEEPING. Perhaps it is because I *do* know this that I am able to look so objectively at the future.

Of course, no matter your attitude, being displaced from your home can cause feelings of insecurity. But there is a lot of work and coordination involved in making your own home environment safe. Did you notice in the previous chapter how many services had to be combined to create a safe and fulfilling existence to age in place at home? So, what are your other options? In this chapter I will discuss senior apartments and subsidized senior housing, assisted living and board and care facilities, continuing care retirement communities (CCRCs) as well as livin' in a whole 'nuther country (that is not a editing or spelling error; it is *affect*).

Senior Apartments and Subsidized Senior Housing

If you are 55 or over, there are many senior communities where you can live. Some of these are simply apartment complexes or retirement hotels. Others are micro-cities, communities that attract those who want a "lifestyle," replete with learning and volunteering opportunities, swimming, dancing, music, clubs, excursions, fitness, and cooking. You can actually own your own unit in some of these communities, which are perfect for those who are not frail or disabled by chronic illness. They are truly communities for active adults. There are no built-in health services or in-home care services provided to residents as part of the rental fees or homeowners' dues. Some do have health care centers, featuring full-service pharmacies, on-site clinical laboratories, radiology and physical therapy services, and a host of specialized medical practice areas available on-site, but access is not included in the typical monthly fees of $800 to $5,000 a month.

For those of you who cannot afford this lifestyle but want to live among your own age group, there are federal and state programs that help pay for housing for some older people with low to moderate incomes. Some of these housing programs also offer help with meals and other activities like house-keeping, shopping, and doing the laundry. Residents usually live in their own apartments in a complex, and rent payments are typically a percentage of your income. There are also senior housing complexes subsidized for low income seniors by the U.S. Department of Housing and Urban Development (HUD). Keep in mind that depending on the area of the country, waiting lists can take years, so it's a good idea to plan well in advance for this option. The official HUD site for senior housing information includes many links with details about various types of housing (visit www.hud.gov and type "seniors" into the search box).

Assisted Living

If your decision to move is based on an imminent or immediate need for assistance with activities of daily living, then assisted living facilities (licensed to care for six or more residents) and board and care homes (limited to six beds) are good options.

Assisted living is in vogue. About 1 million Americans make their homes in assisted living or residential care communities, including about 131,000 who receive assistance under the Medicaid program.[149] The "typical" assisted living resident is 83 years old, and most are women—on average, assisted living resi-dences have 74 percent women and 26 percent men. According to the National Center for Assisted Living, the average assisted living residence ranges from three to 200 units, with an average of 43. The average number of residents in each facility is 40, with a range of one to 175.

Many of my clients ask me about how to choose the right facility. Because so many questions abound, I recently wrote a nine-part newsletter series for my subscribers on assisted living, and I will share some of what I wrote with you now. I will dedicate quite a bit of this chapter to helping you find the right facility, addressing issues of cost, location, and the actual and projected level of care.

Please know that I see these facilities through a lens created from experiences that are likely, in many ways, similar to your own. My mother hated the rock and roll that I listened to growing up (and still listen to). To her, the only true music was classical. However, in my mind, the music of Jethro Tull, The Rolling Stones, The Beatles, Pink Floyd, Led Zeppelin and The Who *is* classical music—it is classic rock. I wanted to listen to that then, I still do, and I will in the future. The music that is currently played in assisted living facilities will not warm my heart when I reach 80. I expect that you may be the same.

Do not delude yourself into thinking you will be immune from suffering the trials and tribulations your parents and grandparents have endured. Grab your albums, eight tracks, medallions, and "right on" mentality, and read on.

The Development of the Assisted Living Model

Just as it was with nursing homes, I think it is important (and interesting) to first understand how this model of long-term care evolved. As we saw earlier, after 1965, many homes for the aged converted to nursing facilities with encouragement from state governments. What we now call assisted living developed on an improvised basis as a reaction to rumors of mistreatment in nursing homes. Many seniors rejected the idea of nursing homes altogether—with their attendant hospital-like designs and operations—and demanded more home-like environments. There were, however, practical obstacles associated with the conversion of existing homes to certified nursing facilities. Some could not meet the regulatory standards even for the lesser level of care (then known as intermediate care) and some simply did not aspire to offer health-related services.

One particular senior who did not want to tolerate the clinical environment of a nursing home was the mother of a woman who is now universally accepted as a pioneer in this industry. Keren Brown Wilson, Ph.D., was repeatedly asked by her mother—who had suffered a debilitating stroke—why she couldn't live in her own place without having to be woken at certain times for her meals. She wanted her own temperature controls in her own room and she wanted the luxury of throwing her back issues of magazines away according to her own timetable. With her daughter in school studying to be a gerontologist, she queried, "Why don't you do something to help people like me?"[150] Her mother's discontent during the following 10 years informed Wilson's ideas for new models of housing and services.[151]

For nearly 30 years, Dr. Brown participated in the history of assisted living on a variety of levels: as a consumer and advocate on behalf of her mother; as an assisted living administrator, owner, and developer; as a consultant on assisted living to state governments; as the chief executive officer of a publicly held company; as an educator; and as a researcher. According to her research, in the early 1980s, developers and operators of assisted living models worked in isolation from one another and approached the industry with different philosophies. She calls these the East Coast and West Coast models, as they began to proliferate in Virginia and Oregon, respectively.

These two models formed the genesis of the hybrid model of assisted living that we see today. Both models were considered novel and controversial by the likes of licensing agencies, nursing facility providers, industry professionals, and advocate groups, all of whom openly talked of their potential to be unlicensed nursing facilities. They had some common elements, such as a commitment to a philosophy of consumer autonomy and an environment that enhanced everyday life. But they also differed in how and to whom they delivered services.

The most historically significant difference has to do with how these new facilities were financed, as the source of funding dictated the types of services offered and the manner in which those services could be delivered. The East Coast model expanded though *private investment money*, under the radar of seemingly disinterested state policy makers. The proprietors focused on financial feasibility, development, standardized training, and communities that resembled large Victorian style bed and breakfasts with sizeable congregate spaces.

The West Coast model affirmatively sought *state policy involvement* with additional care and service capacity. That model was highlighted by a desire to develop an array of long-term care options subsidized by the government so that rich and poor alike could reap the benefits. The availability of public financing for these facilities played a vital role in building apartment-style service models in Oregon. As a prerequisite to obtaining funds, these facilities were required to feature units with locking doors, kitchens, baths, and separate temperature controls. This new model proved attractive to private-pay consumers, and they proliferated.

The first written use of the term "assisted living" was in a 1985 proposal to the state of Oregon. The proposal was for a pilot study of a program that would cover services for 20 nursing home-level Medicaid recipients in a new residential setting. Soon after, the term was being bantered around at presentations and in early trade publications. By 1991, studies included assisted living as an explicit subset of residential care. In 1992, AARP commissioned a national study of assisted living, which was the first to propose a working definition of the term: a group residential setting not licensed as a nursing facility that provides or arranges personal care to meet functional requirements and routine nursing services.[152]

Between 1994 and 1996, assisted living companies began to go public. With access to new capital, they had a corresponding mandate to grow. This initial influx of company offerings inspired changes in strategy for private nursing facility companies. Soon, they began to add dementia care to their *carte du jour*. In 1997, *Fortune* magazine identified assisted living as one of the top three potential growth industries. Before you knew it, every company that provided care to seniors seemed to be calling itself "assisted living." As Wilson herself noted, "With a general desire to adopt the name, suddenly assisted living was a redecorated wing of a nursing facility, or a 16-bed boarding home looking to attract private-pay clients, or congregate housing with dots on the door to identify who got assistance with their medications, or independent living units where residents contracted with home health agencies to provide services."[153]

In contrast to nursing homes, with their extensive federal rules and mandates, the federal government exercises minimal oversight of assisted living facilities. Currently, each state establishes and enforces its own licensing standards for these institutions. More than two-thirds of states use the licensure term "assisted living," while others use titles such as:

- Community-Based Retirement Facilities
- Personal Care
- Adult Congregate Living Care
- Board and Care
- Adult Living Facilities

- Supported Care
- Enhanced Care
- Adult Homes
- Sheltered Housing
- Retirement Residences
- Adult Foster Care
- Residential Care Facilities

Regulation of Assisted Living Facilities

A 2002 study of assisted living policies in each of the 50 states and the District of Columbia showed that states differ in the facilities included under their assisted living regulations based on facility size, services provided, and whether or not the facilities offer specific types of accommodations (e.g., private apartments). In addition, the study found that many states incorporate a distinctive philosophy of care in their regulation of assisted living facilities in order to emphasize residents' choice, independence, dignity, and privacy. Specifically, 28 states have included an assisted living philosophy statement in their regulations, though the particulars of the statements vary.[154] Understanding whether your state's philosophy, as theoretically adopted by its facilities, is consistent with yours may be the decisive factor in whether you or your loved one would be comfortable living in an assisted living environment.

The website of the U.S Department of Health and Human Services Agency for Healthcare Research and Quality (www.ahrq.gov) includes state-specific summaries that identify which agency is responsible for issuing regulations and licensing, and for providing oversight of licensed facilities. Each summary describes the state's approach to regulation and survey practices and special initiatives. Each also has a section on communicating with consumers that describes the information available on the websites of licensing agencies and aging agencies. The websites of the Assisted Living Federation of

America (www.alfa.org) and the National Center for Assisted Living (www.ahcancal.org) go one step further by proffering the regulations verbatim.

A good example of the type of information you can glean from perusing these sites relates to how medications are managed in assisted living facilities. Although all states require facilities to provide some degree of supervision with respect to medications, they differ in the degree to which facility staff can be directly involved in administering them to residents. For example, in some states, unlicensed, nonprofessional staff can administer medications to residents if they have appropriate authorization, training, and general supervision. In others, only staff specifically licensed or certified to administer medications may do so. And in still other states, including California, staff may not administer medications to residents but may only assist residents in taking the medication themselves.

Unfortunately, these websites will not give you information on the *performance* of any facility, nor will any other website or periodical. There is no Five-Star rating system and no national database on abuse and neglect statistics in assisted living facilities. In fact, the problems of residential care settings other than nursing homes have not been well studied or quantified.

We do have a number of inspection reports and media articles that offer up stories of inadequate care.[155] For example, according to a *USA TODAY* analysis of inspection records on assisted living facilities in seven states, more than one in 10 facilities had been cited for neglecting to obtain criminal background checks on employees, as is required by many states.[156] Other research has shown that the same types of problems occur across both assisted living facilities and nursing homes. In one study, 15 percent of the residential care facility staff interviewed reported witnessing other staff members engage in some form of abuse.[157] And several studies have suggested that, like in nursing homes, assisted living facility residents face problems of inadequate care and neglect.[158] The largest data set available relates to ombudsman complaints. According to data from the U.S. Administration on Aging, in 2002 there were 208,762 nursing home ombudsman complaints, compared to 49,463 assisted living ombudsman complaints.

Please do not be lulled into a false sense of security that no abuse takes place in these facilities. Keep in mind that, except for the cognitively compromised, most people in assisted living facilities are the healthy old and they do not require the same level of care that is required for frail nursing home residents. Hence, there is simply less opportunity for neglect. Moreover, there is considerable variation in ombudsman involvement in assisted living, depending on state policies and the resources available to address the myriad complaints that they receive from all types of long-term care facilities. With these caveats in mind, it is useful to know that among the top categories of complaint for assisted living were discharges, billing charges, staffing shortages, and resident care and safety issues.[159]

How to Choose an Assisted Living Facility

While these research findings are a tool in your cache, you cannot simply rely on ombudsman complaints or the lack thereof as a barometer of how these facilities are performing as a whole. They do provide a small window into the current state of assisted living facilities, but they do not tell the whole story. And experts opine that the challenges faced by these types of facilities will only increase as demand rises and the care needs of the residents grow increasingly complex.

Further compounding the difficulty of evaluating specific facilities is the lack of uniform standards across states. This has resulted in variations in monitoring quality-of-care and consumer protection issues, making it difficult if not impossible to uniformly identify and report industry wide problems, let alone particular incidents at specific facilities. I would *not* recommend reliance on an inspection report to ascertain anything about a particular facility. True, all states conduct periodic inspections or surveys of facilities to ensure that they comply with licensing requirements. But they vary in frequency and content and in the range of enforcement mechanisms that can be used to correct problems. Some state licensing agencies are required to inspect facilities annually, while others are required to inspect facilities every 15 months or every two years. In California, inspections must take place every five years.

We do know, however, that as with the nursing home industry, it is very challenging to attract and keep qualified staff in assisted living facilities. But unlike in the nursing home industry, requirements for staff levels, qualifications, and training vary among the states. In some, regulations require facilities to maintain a minimum number of full-time staff based on the total number of residents, while in others the number of staff must only be sufficient to meet the needs of residents. In still other states, there is no guidance at all on how large the staff must be to provide for the residents' needs.

It goes without saying that ensuring that properly trained (non-criminal) assisted living caregivers are in place is important. By the same token, actually having *enough* on the job is critical. Nonetheless, inspection records from the seven states analyzed by *USA TODAY* show that facilities were repeatedly cited for having too few caregivers on duty. They were likewise cited for their outright failure to have administrators on site to oversee less experienced caregivers or to pitch in on days of low staffing. These findings are consistent with the results of a 1999 report by the

General Accounting Office, in which inadequate training, insufficient staffing, high turnover, and low pay were blamed for the most common quality of care problems.

Again, just as with nursing homes, one of the most important indicators of whether a facility is good enough for you is how long the staff members have been there. And although less important in assisted living facilities, it is still true that the higher the ratio of staff to residents, the more likely an individual's needs will not be ignored. It also is evidence of a philosophy of care that puts a resident's comfort above profits. If there is no mandated staff ratio and the levels at one facility are significantly higher than at a neighboring facility, I would naturally gravitate toward the former.

I believe that as long as you understand what to look for and what to demand, assisted living is a very good option for you if you cannot stay in your own home. If you are charting a course in this direction, you first need to visit a facility and "feel it." The focus should be on the facility's services rather than the attractiveness of the building itself. Some have lavish furnishings (particularly in the lobby) but show little interest in the well-being of their residents. That said, a facility's appearance does have some significance, and particularly important are the residents' rooms. If residents can furnish and decorate their own rooms, the facility will feel more like a home. If, on the other hand, all rooms have the same institutional decor, residents are more likely to feel depressed and/or dissatisfied.

Next, you need to learn about facility services, costs, and policies that will impact your experience. Most of my clients are faced with choosing an assisted living facility without having the key information they need in order to identify the one most likely to meet their individual needs, and my review of the GAO report leads me to believe that this is a national phenomenon. Information about staffing levels and qualifications, costs and potential cost increases, and the circumstances that could lead to involuntary discharge from the facility are consistently withheld from the consumer.[160] Also, consumers are often presented with incomplete and inaccurate information.

According to the GAO, family members often have difficulty grasping information that is presented to them about care options, especially when decisions must be made quickly to address a crisis situation. Under these circumstances, you may not know what questions to ask or how to assess and compare the responses that you receive in order to identify the facility that can best meet your individual needs. A likely consequence is that the you or your loved one will have to move again within a short time, which is very stressful and can have extensive psychological and health ramifications.

Let's look at why signing an assisted living agreement is so vastly different from entering into a simple residential lease. Assisted living is often promoted as supporting the concept of "aging in place," which allows residents to remain in a facility as their health conditions decline or their needs change. The ability of residents to age in place is reflected in a facility's admission and discharge criteria or its rules governing who it will permit to move in and when they may be required to leave. However, there is also considerable variation across states in admission and discharge criteria, some of which results from regulatory limits on allowable conditions or services in assisted living facilities, the facilities' choice of who to serve, and the particular services they choose to provide or make available.

Most facilities are required to conduct an initial assessment and create a care plan to determine the services to be provided to you prior to admission. These include your medical condition, mental capacity, personal preferences, and ability to carry

out routine daily tasks. A similar meeting usually occurs whenever there is a significant change in your condition, or at least
once every twelve months, to ensure that the written care plan
is kept up-to-date. Only some facilities will admit or retain you
if you require assistance to transfer from bed to chair or wheelchair, and some will not admit or retain you if you have
moderate to severe cognitive problems.

Regardless of the requirement to conduct an annual assessment,
an assisted living facility must be aware of changes in your physical,
mental, or emotional condition. Significant changes in health must
be reported to your doctor and (if applicable) to a close family
member or friend. Moreover, assessments must be updated
frequently enough to maintain accuracy. At minimum, the updates
must include physical setbacks and emotional traumas (the death
of a family member, for instance). Here in California, regulations
contain a list of services that facility staff are generally not allowed
to provide, including catheter care, colostomy care, and injections.
Other states limit skilled nursing care to residents who need it only
on a part-time, intermittent basis and restrict it to no more than
120 days per year. Still others have no explicit restrictions on the
types or levels of care that facility staff can provide.

When you do not receive adequate information before selecting
an assisted living facility, you are less likely to find a facility that
can satisfactorily address your personal and ever-changing care
needs. What happens if your condition changes after living in
your apartment for six years? Will you be able to remain in what
you have come to call home? What happens if you are stricken
with Alzheimer's disease or your spouse—with whom you share
an apartment and have shared a life—is diagnosed with dementia?
How will the facility handle it? *Can* they handle it?

Many of my clients heavily rely on facility information that
they receive in various ways, including marketing brochures. This

rarely clarifies anything and that is why they call me for sugges-tions. In 1999, the GAO reported that marketing materials, contracts, and other written materials that facilities give consumers were often vague, incomplete, or misleading. Specifically, facilities' written materials often did not contain key information, such as a description of services not covered or not available at the facility, the staff's qualifications and training, circumstances under which costs might change, assistance residents would receive with medication administration, facility practices in assessing needs, or criteria for discharging residents.[161]

This lack of clear information is still a problem. In response to consumers' continued difficulty obtaining full disclosure of the information they need,[162] 18 states have instituted information disclosure policies, including requirements for the use of uniform disclosure statements or for the contents of written materials provided to prospective residents.[163] Nevertheless, it is important that you know that things you have read in brochures and other adver-tising information from the provider may not show up in your contract. Check them against each other to be sure that any adver-tised service you want is included in the actual resident agreement. Likewise, you should be wary of admission agreements that are vague in explaining when extra charges are assessed. For example, some admission agreements set out price levels that give the facility a great deal of discretion in deciding when your care needs may warrant a price increase. If an admission agreement does not provide for varying rates, try to get a commitment in writing as to when and under what circumstances the rates will change.

What Do I Get for My Money?

According to the National Investment Center's *Investment Guide 2010*, the median monthly rate for assisted living communities is $3,326 per month. This covers room and board, basic utilities (electricity, heat, water, and garbage), basic housekeeping (including fresh linens), and some meals. Many facilities include 20 to 40 meals as part of the monthly package. The cost of senior programming and activities is also typically included in this price. Most facilities have very active calendars of social events.

Most facilities charge money on top of the base rate to assist individuals with activities of daily living (ADLs). Some charge these fees based on a point system, with points assigned according to how many items one needs assistance with. A facility might use a numeric system from one to three or five, based on the number of ADLs. The levels of care might be described as minimal, moderate, or maximal, or as care assist or care enhanced. I met with the executive directive of a facility that bases fees on how much time it takes staff to assist the resident with their ADLs. Most also have additional charges for medications, personal hygiene, and medical supplies

Regardless of the facility's practice, it is important to understand that this *à la carte* method of assigning levels of care with fee increments of $300–$400 for each level can add up to as much as $4,000 in additional monthly costs, especially if an individual has Alzheimer's disease, since the manpower and extra training required of those who care for these afflicted residents goes beyond simple assistance with bathing and grooming. Some facilities are exclusively dedicated to caring for those with the disease and some have specialized neighborhoods or communities within their facilities on a separate floor.

I have found most facilities to be very forthcoming in explaining their fee structures thoroughly so there will be no surprises later. It is in the best interest of the facility and the potential resident to do so. Importantly, while the facility can charge whatever the market will bear, the rates must be stated in the admission agreement. Despite this transparency, **pay special**

attention to all up-front fees! Some facilities call these "administrative fees," "community fees," or "application fees," and they can range from $250 to $5,000. In some states, facilities are permitted to charge for such pre-admission fees if they are clearly stated in the admission agreement. Ask what each fee covers and find out under what circumstances they can be refunded. For example, if you do not enter the facility, or if the facility does not perform an appraisal (assessment), or fails to provide a written disclosure of the pre-admission fee charges and refund conditions, you may be able to demand a proportional refund of pre-admission fees.

One of the most important pieces of information to find out is how long your bed will be held if you have a lengthy hospital stay or a vacation. If your contract does not include a bed-hold policy—both for unavoidable absences (such as hospitalizations or recuperation in rehabilitation settings) and optional absences (such as vacations, visits to family, etc.)—ask what their policy is. It must include the conditions under which the facility will hold your bed, what this costs, who must pay for it, and the circumstances under which your bed will no longer be held. Assisted living facilities are accepting people with higher and higher levels of chronic illnesses and dementia and, as a result, residents may go to the hospital many times over during the course of residency. This makes the bed-hold policy very important. When helping my clients find the right facilities for themselves or their loved ones, I always ask whether any fees are stopped or reduced when the resident is away from the home. Changes in fees for special circumstances should be a part of your assisted living contract.

If you do not have a family member or a friend to accompany you to the doctor, you need to know whether transportation is provided or whether the facility will help arrange for outside transportation. Also important is a contractual commitment for how often health care professionals—nurses, doctors, therapists, etc.—come to the facility. The contract should specify what kinds of health services will be provided by staff, such as helping with medications, calling in prescriptions to the pharmacy, or arranging for prescription delivery. Many facilities have a pharmacy that they prefer, and that pharmacy may or may not take specific prescription discount plans. Ask the provider about options for getting prescriptions, so that medication costs do not increase.

Medicare does not pay for assisted living. There is, however, limited assistance from other sources for low-income persons. If you qualify for SSI (Supplemental Security Income) and State Supplemental Payment (SSP), state regulations may limit how much the facility can charge you each month. Although fewer and fewer facilities are willing to take the low payment rate, if you have low personal care needs, some facilities may be more willing to admit you on SSI/SSP. In some states, Medicaid (the state program for low income seniors) pays for assisted living care, adult family home care, in-home care, and/or nursing home placement. In others, Medicaid pays for these services through waivers, which are vehicles states can use to test new or existing ways to deliver and pay for health care services. States can apply for home and community-based waivers to provide long-term care services outside of institutional settings. The issue is access: Since the state reimburses providers much less than they can earn from private pay clients, many are reluctant to accept Medicaid residents at all.

If you would like to know if your state has a Medicaid waiver program, visit the Medicaid website (www.medicaid.gov). *Caveat emptor*, however:

I had the unfortunate experience of having to advocate for a woman who was evicted from a facility after living there for 12 years when she ran out of money. She was 99 years old. She had been promised that when her funds ran out she could convert to Medicaid and remain at the community. Turns out, when the time came, the community said they were at their limit for Medicaid residents and told her to either continue paying privately or find a new assisted living community.

There are several terms you may see included in discussions of payment for assisted living. For example, a "continuing care contract" can require you to pay a lump sum of money in exchange for a stay of over one year. A "life care contract" (which is a particular type of continuing care contract) can require you to pay all or most of your savings in exchange for residence in certain facilities for the remainder of your life. An assisted living facility can offer a life care contract only if the facility operates an adjacent nursing home. The life care contract must offer you all necessary levels of care, including nursing home care. Many life care contracts are offered by facilities associated with religious denominations or non-profit organizations. Most often you see these types of agreements in continuing care retirement communities, which are discussed below.

It is important to understand that, however the bill is being footed, often there is a separate document to be signed by someone else who will take responsibility for payment for your care. They may be referred to as a "responsible party," "authorized representative," "agent for resident," or by some other similar term. If your friend or family member does not want to use their own funds to pay for your care, any document they sign should say that they are responsible "only to the extent of the resident's personal funds and/or resources." This means that they will not be required to use their own money for your care, but rather they will simply be responsible for ensuring that your resources are used in a timely manner to pay all bills. This rule should be applied to any nursing home contract as well!

Board and Care

Board and care homes are group living arrangements with six beds or less, designed to meet the needs of people who cannot live independently but who do not need nursing home services. A residential or board and care home is usually a converted house where the caregiver is a homeowner or single proprietor with little or no support staff. Most board and care homes provide help with some of the activities of daily living such as bathing, dressing, and using the bathroom. Some also house Alzheimer's patients. Board and care homes are sometimes called "group homes."

Many of these homes do not get payment from Medicare or Medicaid. The difference in licensing is usually based on the size of the facility or the services it can offer. The cost for board and care homes is typically much less than for large, new, apartment-style assisted living facilities. In your search for a suitable board and care facility, you will need to pay attention to the same items that you focus on in your quest for assisted living and, as I discuss next, continuing care retirement communities.

Continuing Care Retirement Communities

Continuing care retirement communities (CCRCs) are retirement communities with more than one kind of housing and different levels of care. They are generally on large campuses, and where you live depends on the level of care you need. In the same community, there may be individual homes or apartments for residents who still live on their own, an assisted living facility for people who need some help with daily care, and a nursing home for those who require higher levels of care. Residents move from one level to another based on their needs, but they stay within the CCRC.

Not-for-profit organizations, often with faith-based affiliations and/or that cater to affinity groups, still sponsor the majority of CCRCs. Only about 18 percent of the CCRCs currently in operation have for-profit ownership. Approximately half of all CCRCs are affiliated with faith-based organizations; among those affiliations, 21 percent are Lutheran, 18 percent are Methodist, 14 percent are Presbyterian, and 13 percent are Roman Catholic.[164]

CCRCs are not regulated by the federal government; 38 states have some level of regulation specifically addressing CCRCs, while 12 states plus the District of Columbia do not. Among the 38 states that do have regulations, CCRCs are overseen by a variety of state departments. Where there is oversight, it is through one of a number of departments. Because of the unique financial relationship between the resident and the CCRC, some states oversee these communities through departments that concentrate on insurance, financial services, or banking. Still other states regulate them through departments one would more logically associate with caring for the elderly, such as social services, aging or elder services, or community affairs.

By definition, a CCRC must provide skilled care to residents who need it. Their nursing homes, like any free-standing nursing home, are subject to federal oversight if they participate in Medicare or Medicaid programs. Therefore, if you are considering a CCRC, be sure to check the record of its nursing home. Your CCRC contract usually requires you to use the CCRC's nursing home if you need this level of care. Some CCRCs will only admit your into their nursing home if you have previously lived in another section of the retirement community, such as assisted living or an independent area. Other CCRCs may admit you into their nursing home facilities as if they were stand-alone facilities, and have you pay the nursing home per diem or market rate. Other CCRCs may temporarily admit you directly into assisted living or nursing facilities to broaden their customer base and to generate revenue.

Most if not all CCRCs require a large payment—called an entry fee—before you move in. It is not unusual for these to fees to range from $100,000 to $1 million. CCRCs also charge monthly fees to cover housing and convenience services, and these typically range from $3,000 to $5,000, but may increase as needs change. As a prospective resident, you must submit detailed financial information that includes income and tax records to ensure that you can pay the fees over time. The up-front sum is used to prepay for care as well as to provide the facility money to operate. Therein lies the rub: Entering a CCRC often means committing a large portion of your assets.

CCRCs typically offer one of three general types of contracts involving different combinations of entrance and monthly fee payments. Some CCRCs will offer you a choice of contract type, while others may offer only one.

> **Extensive or Life Care Contracts (TYPE A):** These contracts include housing, residential services, and amenities—including unlimited use of health care services—at little or no increase in monthly fees as you move from independent living to assisted living, and, if needed, to nursing care. They characteristically feature substantial entrance fees but may be attractive because monthly payments do not increase significantly as you move through the different levels of care. In this scenario, the CCRC absorbs the risk of any increases in the cost of providing your health and long-term care.

> **Modified Contracts (TYPE B):** These contracts offer lower monthly fees than the life care contracts and include the same housing and residential services, but only include some health care services in the initial monthly rate.

Should your needs exceed that level of services, the fees increase to market rates. This can create uncertainty, as there is no way to predict what the market daily rate or discounted daily rate (as determined by the CCRC) will be for future assisted living or nursing care utilization.

Fee-for-Service Contract (TYPE C): These contracts include the same housing, residential services, and amenities as the previous two contractual arrangements but require you to pay market rates for all health-related services on an as-needed basis. While paying as you go as an independent resident may involve lower entrance and monthly fees, you also absorb the risk of higher long-term care expenses.

Rental Agreements: Some CCRCs, but not many, offer rental agreements, which generally require no entrance fees but guarantee access to CCRC services and health care. Others offer benevolence care. For many CCRCs, providing support for residents who qualify for financial assistance or who run out of funds is viewed as a fulfillment of the organization's mission and purpose. These CCRCs will typically evaluate your financial status in order to project the financial resources that may be required to meet your potential financial shortfall. This type of financial aid could also be a critical expense area for which a CCRC must plan in order to protect the financial health of the entire community.

The large majority of these contracts offer some type of entrance fee refund at death or move-out. This may include a traditional declining-scale feature (where the refund/repayment declines over time), a partial refund/repayment, or, in some cases, a full refund/repayment. A declining-scale refund feature, for example, may reduce the entrance fee refund by 2 percent per month, with a one-time 4 percent administration fee; after 48 months of residency, the refund is reduced to zero. Many CCRCs, however, offer contracts that refund a specific percentage of the entrance fees regardless of the length of residency; for example, several communities currently offer 100, 90, 75, or 50 percent refundable contracts. Also, an individual CCRC may offer one or more refund options. Any refund or repayment due is paid to you if the contract is terminated or to your estate upon your death; however, the timing of the refund or repayment will vary. It is often paid only after your apartment or cottage is reoccupied.[165]

These contracts can be very complicated and lengthy. Some states require that CCRC license applicants submit a copy of the contract form to be entered into with residents as part of the licensure process. In some of those states the contract form must be approved by the state, while in others contracts are simply required to be legible or written in clear and understandable language. Of the 38 states with CCRC-specific licensure laws, 30 require that CCRC contracts include a provision that confers a "cooling off" period in which you would have the right to cancel your contract and receive a full refund of entrance fees, less certain costs. The prescribed periods during which such cancellation rights may be exercised range from prior-to-occupancy to as long as one year after occupancy, and they allow you to exit your contract without penalty or forfeiture of previously paid funds.

CCRCs are a brilliant option if you can afford the price of entry and want to have access to housing and health care in a single community as you age. In fact, according to the American Association of Homes and Services for the Aging, at least 745,000 older adults live in such communities. A survey conducted by American Seniors Housing Association (ASHA) and published in the organization's *Independent Living Report, 2009* identified the following financial demographic characteristics of CCRC residents: They have a net worth ranging from less than $50,000 to $2 million, and at least half reported a total net worth of $300,000 or more. Only 8 percent of those living in entrance-fee CCRCs reported a net worth of less than $100,000, compared to 25 percent of those in rental CCRCs; 32 percent of those living in entrance-fee CCRCs had a net worth of $1 million or more, compared to 14 percent for those in rental CCRCs.

The financial risks faced by the CCRC industry were explored in a 2010 GAO report. The disquiet was solvency centric and included concerns that:

- Residents could lose the refundable portion of their entrance fees—which may amount to hundreds of thousands of dollars or more—if a CCRC encounters financial difficulties or goes bankrupt.
- Residents could face greater-than-expected increases in monthly or other fees that could erode their existing assets or make the CCRC unaffordable to them.
- Some residents might experience "buyer's remorse" after entering a CCRC if the community, services, or other aspects of the CCRC do not match their initial perceptions. If they wish to move, they might find that the contractually designated rescission period has ended, resulting in significant fines or reductions to the refundable portion of their entrance fees.
- Residents might face the risk of being transferred involuntarily from one level of care to another, or of not being able to obtain on-site assisted living or nursing care when needed. The latter could prove to be

extremely stressful as it presents a threat to individual autonomy.[166]

The nonprofit entities that run CCRCs can issue tax-exempt bonds through cooperative local government agencies for funding. As of February 29, 2012, 2 percent of bonds tied to these communities were in default, the sixth highest of 46 types of municipal debt.[167] While CCRC bankruptcies have been rare, and few residents have lost their housing or their entrance fees, a CCRC collapse could put you in a difficult financial situation. This is a legitimate concern, especially in the current down economy. Many people sell their homes to pay the steep entrance fees, but homes are not selling, which suppresses occupancy levels; the longer people put off buying into facilities, the more frail they become and the more costly their care. This places financial stress on the CCRC, which is then forced to raise monthly fees, move people into different areas on campus with different profit centers, or fail.

Some states affirmatively attempt to protect the financial interests of CCRC residents by (1) establishing requirements for fees and deposits to be escrowed, (2) addressing criteria for monthly fee increases, or (3) placing liens on CCRC assets on behalf of residents or conferring a preferred status on resident claims to such assets in the event of liquidation.[168]

Since your life savings and your legacy intentions could be impacted by a community's financial viability, I strongly recommend that you (or a competent advisor on your behalf) investigate any CCRC's financial fitness by looking at its audited financial statements. Look for:

- Days of cash on hand, and compare it to that of other facilities (CCRCs with one campus average 306 days of cash on hand; those with multiple sites average 281);
- The cash-to-debt figure (which should be about 35%);
- Details on any bond financing and whether the facility

is meeting the terms (typically, banks require 300 days of cash on hand and a minimum of 25 percent cash to debt);[169]

- The source of cash for running the day-to-day operations. If the CCRC relies heavily on investment income, donations or entry fees, this may signify an inability to run on income from operations and impending financial doom;
- The occupancy rate, since a facility with a higher occupancy rate is less likely to look to you to re-coup operating expenses. I always ask the administrator about the census. Ideally, you want to see that the facility is almost completely occupied.

You can find out if a CCRC is accredited and get advice on selecting this type of community from the Continuing Care Accreditation Commission, either by telephone (202-783-7286) or on the web (www.ccaconline.org). You can also call the agency that regulates CCRCs in your state and investigate the complaint history of any community.

A Special Note About Alzheimer's and Dementia Care

Just last night, I told someone that I like being concise when I speak. The truth is, I wanted to say succinct, but that word did not come to me until this morning. When it came, I felt like I gave birth. That word was there, waiting all night, germinating and gestating to fall from my tongue. It was a horrible feeling not to be able to conjure a word that is an ordinary part of my vocabulary. I am 49 years old and this happens to me all too often. Am I getting Alzheimer's disease? Do you ever wonder if you are on the precipice of developing this disease?

When someone truly loses their memory, it is like a glass slipping from their hand. As they try to retrieve it from the abyss of synaptic failure, a hallmark of Alzheimer's disease, it shatters and leaves in its wake a feeling of distress and helplessness. The thought dies because the neuron upon which it relied dies.

There are many age-associated memory problems that can change your ability to think or remember. It is important to differentiate normal aging and treatable causes of memory loss from irreversible causes such as dementia. Some of the signs and symptoms to watch for are: increasing and persistent forgetfulness (repeating the same questions or forgetting conversations, appointments, and dates); difficulty with familiar and complex tasks (e.g., balancing a checkbook or preparing a meal; orientation (time and dates); language (e.g., difficulty with word finding and naming objects); reasoning ability (poor judgment and decision making); personality and behavior changes (increased irritability, apathy, and restlessness).

The truth is that Alzheimer's is an old person's disease. Five percent of the age 65 population has Alzheimer's disease, and 50 percent of the population over 85 has it. Individuals with cognitive impairments are increasingly finding their homes in assisted living facilities. As of 2005, 26 percent of assisted living residents with dementia were moderately impaired and 61 percent were severely impaired.[170] Others (26 percent) have psychiatric disturbances such as depression or anxiety disorders.[171] Some reports indicate that behavioral symptoms affect 34 percent of all assisted living residents,[172] and 56 percent of those with dementia.[173]

Mild cognitive impairment (MCI) is an intermediate stage between the expected cognitive decline of normal aging and the more pronounced decline of dementia. It involves problems with memory, language, thinking, and judgment that are greater than typical age-related changes. If you have MCI, you may be aware that your memory or mental function has "slipped." Family and close friends may also notice changes. Generally these changes are not severe enough to interfere with day-to-day life and usual activities. Mild cognitive impairment increases your risk of later developing dementia, including Alzheimer's disease, especially when your main difficulty is with memory. Some people with mild cognitive impairment never get worse, and a few eventually get better, and because MCI does not always result in Alzheimer's disease, those individuals may never experience a disturbance in their surroundings.

When a resident or prospective resident has Alzheimer's disease or some other form of dementia, an assisted living facility can admit or retain them only if it complies with dementia-specific regulations regarding staffing, training, fire safety, and other safety measures. Although, as we learned, there are no uniform industry regulations, all states require an annual medical assessment, adequate supervision, enhanced physical plant safety, and an appropriate activity program. And while state-determined regulations are rapidly changing to better ensure that dementia-related care needs are met, standards for medication use and review, staff preparation and training related to individualized approaches, and use of person-centered programs of care too often lag behind.[174]

The Assisted Living Workgroup (ALW) was formed to develop recommendations for assisted living on a national scale. It was a national initiative of nearly 50 organizations—representing providers, consumers, long-term care and health care professionals, and regulators, among others—that joined forces at the behest of the U.S. Senate Special Committee on Aging. Its final report, published in 2003, notes that it is important to find facilities for Alzheimer's patients that provide structured routines. According to the ALW, assisted living communities that accommodate special care residents should provide daily interactions and experiences that are meaningful (based upon residents' interests, feelings, and lifestyle), appropriate (for their abilities and functioning levels), and respectful (of residents' age, beliefs, cultures, values, and life experiences), as determined by individual assessments and as indicated in their service plans.[175] I tell my clients to pay attention to how much time the staff takes to gather specific lifestyle information about their loved ones in order to individually cater to his/her needs. This is called person-centered care.[176]

The aim of person-centered care is to acknowledge the personhood of people with Alzheimer's disease in all aspects of their care. It is recognition that the personality of the person with Alzheimer's disease is concealed but not lost; the dementia forms only part of his total identity and the larger part of him continues to be the possession of his own uniqueness. Possessing this rich history allows the staff to effectively empower, reassure, and nurture the person with dementia and form the basis of a positive supportive relationship in which he continues to live life the way he would like to, in the manner in which he is still capable. Decision-making can be directed by the resident or with assistance from family or a designated surrogate decision maker if the resident is unable to fully communicate.

There are unique concerns when residents wander, and a big challenge for assisted living staff is balancing safety with quality of life. Facilities may only use specialized devices to prevent them from leaving the building if certain requirements are met. Delayed egress doors (doors that delay but do not prevent a resident's exit from the building) and locked doors/perimeters require special fire clearances, and locking is only allowed with prior approval from the state's licensing department. Structured wandering opportunities (e.g., enclosed wandering paths or wandering paths in secure outside spaces) may decrease residents' desire to leave their communities unsupervised. The Alzheimer's Association has fashioned guidelines for wandering to address this behavioral challenge. They recommend an evaluation for exit seeking behavior prior to the resident moving in and the development of a service plan that promotes resident choice, mobility, and safety. These mechanisms can manage elopement behavior and create an environment that incorporates features of home rather than institutional life.[177]

German nursing homes have been using a novel approach to stopping Alzheimer's patients from wandering off in the form of phantom bus stops. One facility created an exact replica of a standard stop outside, with one small difference: buses do not use it. The center had been forced to rely on police to retrieve patients who waited for or boarded buses, wanting to return to their often non-existent homes and families. The residents recognize the green and yellow bus sign and remember that waiting there means they will go home. The result is that errant patients now wait for their trip home at the bus stop, before quickly forgetting why they are there in the first place. The staff then approach them and tell them that the bus is coming later and invites them in for a coffee. Within minutes they have completely forgotten they wanted to leave.

Most states mandate that facilities that care for individuals with dementia provide an adequate number of staff to support the physical, social, emotional, safety, and health care needs of each resident with dementia. Facilities must have activity programs that address the needs and limitations of residents with dementia. If a facility advertises or promotes specialized dementia care, it should describe its special dementia-related features in its plan of operation. The admission agreement should inform the resident or his legal representative that the special features are described in the plan of operation, and that the plan of operation is available for review on request.

Every human being has a right to assert his or her needs and wants and pain. For someone with Alzheimer's, what we think of as a simple act of communication can be extremely challenging, however. According to the Alzheimer's Association, effective communication involves allowing residents time to process requests and instructions. Staff must understand behaviors and use methods that the individual can understand, such as gentle touch, direct eye contact, smiles, and a pleasant tone of voice.[178] From my experience, Alzheimer's patients respond better to limited choices than to open-ended questions. The facility should also ensure that special training requirements are met by staff who provide care to residents with dementia, as they need a different skill set. It is a very complex illness with different phases and clinical symptoms; without the most up-to-date skills and knowledge, the staff is at a disadvantage as they try to meet the residents' individual needs, wants, and desires. Always ask what type of special training in managing Alzheimer's disease the staff has and how often they receive training.

Please know that a move for any older adult can cause depression. But for the cognitively compromised, the early days of moving into an assisted living community can be more overwhelming and more intense than for their intact peers. Find out how the community will handle your loved one's anxiety. Above all else, find a place where the staff and administrator exude warmth and love and whose references are impeccable. Together with our children, those who have Alzheimer's disease are the most vulnerable human beings on the planet.

Paying for Long-Term Care

Chapter 11 is devoted entirely to the subject of paying for the various types of long-term care that I have outlined in this and the previous chapter, but I will offer you a short preview here. Prior to January 1, 1997, the cost of long-term care was tax deductible only if the primary reason for an individual's placement in a long-term care facility was medical. If the placement was for personal or family reasons, only that part of the fee that was directly tied to medical services was deductible. In 1996, Congress passed and President Clinton signed the Health Insurance Portability and Accountability Act (HIPAA). According to HIPAA, qualified long-term care services are deductible from gross income as an itemized deduction, subject to the limitation that when added to any other unreimbursed medical expenses for the year, only the amount that exceeds 7.5 percent of adjusted gross income is an itemized deduction.

As a result of HIPAA, maintenance or personal care services that are required by an individual who is unable to perform at least two activities of daily living (eating, bathing, dressing, toileting, ambulating, etc.) or who suffers from severe cognitive impairment, or who requires supervision to protect herself from threats to her own health or safety are deductible as itemized medical expenses *if* those services are provided pursuant to a plan of care prescribed by a licensed health care practitioner. The resident must have been certified within the previous 12 months as "chronically ill" by a licensed health care practitioner.

THAT IS A MOUTHFUL!

What it means is that for assisted living facilities that utilize a licensed health care practitioner (i.e., a registered nurse) to help prepare a plan of care in conjunction with the resident's physician, and for those residents who meet the criteria, it would appear that the entire monthly cost may be deductible. Depending upon your family's specific situation, eligibility for this deduction may create a substantial tax benefit for you or your providers.

Should you have further questions on the tax treatment of assisted living arrangements, please seek the advice of a qualified tax planner or financial advisor.

Hasta La Vista, Baby!

As this chapter has hopefully made clear, you have many options in this country—some better, some worse—when it comes to how you spend your later years. But there is one more choice. You can always leave the country and discard the shackles of impending poverty that bound you to this great nation and its addiction to all things disposable. There are a number of countries that would be happy to take your money and lavish you with basic human needs like food, housing, and health care for a fraction of what you would pay here.

I recently attended the *Los Angeles Times* Travel Show because I heard I could learn about many opportunities to retire outside the country. My husband and I sat though a presentation on Ecuador. I was heartened to hear how the retirement communities there are filled with expatriates; I had previously only associated that country with my favorite scientist, Darwin, and the Galapagos Islands. The same can be said for Uruguay, Belize, the South of France, Panama, and Nicaragua.

These countries are safe and have modern conveniences. You can see a movie on the same day that it opens in the United States for a fraction of the ticket price. There are clinics with the latest technology and university medical schools. In Provençe, France, there is even an Anglo-American group. Apparently, you can live very comfortably for $1,500 a month in many a foreign land. All you need is a little moola, *parlez français*, or *hablas español*.

If you are not ready to completely uproot, there are other ways to take advantage of international resources and see a bit of the world in the process. Medical tourism is the practice of traveling abroad to obtain health care services. Typically you can not only save a substantial amount of money, but also receive world-class service—possibly even *better* than what you would receive here. According to the National Coalition on Health Care, in 2005 more than 500,000 Americans chose offshore medical treatment from places like Thailand, Singapore, and India. Experts predict that by 2012, medical tourism will grow to be a $110 billion business. Even some U.S. employers have begun exploring medical travel programs as a way to cut employee health care costs.

You can keep a high deductible U.S. medical policy and carry an international policy for about $1,000 a year. In the near future I will be traveling to these countries to report on them more thoroughly, and they will be the subject of a forthcoming newsletter. Hopefully, if you haven't already, you will sign up to get my newsletter after reading and enjoying this book.

CHAPTER 9

The Road to Good Health Is Paved with Good Sweat

Do you see that? It is a droplet of sweat, to be followed by many others. If I were not using a computer, the paper would be stained by the sickness I am purging from my pores. I just got back from the gym. I hate exercising. It's not so much that I don't like sweating; I just get bored very easily, of everything. Also, when I see people running I think, *Where the heck are they going?* But, I do not want to have a heart attack or stroke or get Alzheimer's disease. I have too much to live for and I do not want to end up in a nursing home because I became a sick old person.

I wish that I could just reiterate what you have surely heard repeatedly about the connection between healthy lifestyle choices, exercise, and chronic illness and be done with it. But that does not seem to work. We have been bombarded with this information for years, yet so many people are still very obese in this country. So I will outline in very precise terms how staying fit and making the right choices can keep you out of a nursing home. Of course, you could always bypass this hard work and ignore my message. Fall prey to a late night infomercial for weight loss supplements instead. Or, explore the benefits of lap band surgery (which, ironically, Medicare might cover). These are short cuts with varying results, but they are not likely to keep you healthy enough to stay out of long-term care. For that, you can get sweaty for just 20–30 minutes a day and eat your fruits and vegetables.

The main chronic medical conditions associated with nursing home admissions are stroke and dementia.[179] Stroke prevention results in fewer cases admitted to the nursing home, older age at first admission, and a smaller proportion of remaining life spent there.[180] Regular exercise can help protect you from (among other things that are outside the scope of my expertise) stroke and its underlying risk factors such as high blood pressure and noninsulin-dependent diabetes. And because Alzheimer's disease is the second most feared disease in this country next to cancer, you should know that exercise can stave that off too. And the sooner you start, the better, since it is now widely accepted that the disease process starts a good 15 years before the clinical symptoms of Alzheimer's disease rear their ugly head. All of these chronic diseases increase your chances of losing your independence. If this happens, you will be pestered to death by family members, caregivers, and maybe even some government social worker because you will be frail and dependent.

What Is a Stroke?

My friend's father just had a stroke. He is 82. Prior to the stroke he was a very fun-loving, affable man. Now, he is paralyzed and suffering from aphasia (the loss of ability to understand or express speech). In the aging industry, we understandably focus a lot of our energy on Alzheimer's disease, but stroke is the third leading cause of death in the United States, behind high blood pressure and cancer. Every 45 seconds someone in the United States has a stroke and every three minutes someone dies from a stroke.

I got an A+ on my final paper in my physiology of aging class at the University of Southern California on the matter of stroke and the risk factors thereof. I own a mobile ultrasound stroke screening company with my husband, and our sonographers have screened more than 30,000 people over the last 13 years. Also, I have a bachelor of science degree in speech pathology, and I studied the pathology of strokes as an undergraduate. I want to share with you now some of the information I have gathered from my studies and from my experiences with real human beings in our business.

The term *stroke* describes a clinical diagnosis of observed loss of neurologic function due to ischemia following acute loss of circulation.[181] I did that spiel for my professor; I seek to impress. Now, let's talk in real people terms!

Atherosclerosis in the carotid arteries is the main cause of age-related strokes.[182] In atherosclerosis, fatty deposits (ulcerated plaque) build up on the inner walls of the arteries, usually over many years, making older individuals more susceptible to stroke. This plaque is composed of a porridge-like accumulation of cholesterol and their compounds within a fibrous coat that protrudes from the inner lining of the arteries and obstructs blood flow to the brain. The brain requires a constant flow of blood to work properly, and if this flow is disrupted, brain cells do not receive enough oxygen, resulting in cell death; nerve cells in the part of the brain that are deprived of oxygen become dysfunctional.[183] Additionally, plaque accumulation causes injury to the arteries and initiates a process called the inflammatory response. This cycle usually repeats itself, forming atherosclerotic lesions,[184] which results in blood-flow abnormalities and compromised oxygen supply to the target organ, the brain.[185]

Having a stroke is not an inevitable part of aging. In fact, stroke is not just an older person's disease—28 percent of strokes occur in people under the age of 65. That said, it is an *age-related* disease. About 75 percent of stroke cases involve people over the age of 55.[186] And your risk of having a stroke increases with age; in fact, after 55 the incidence of stroke more than doubles in each successive decade.[187]

Stroke is influenced by more than just the number of years you've been on this planet. Some of these—gender, family history, and of course age—are beyond your control. However, you can substantially reduce your overall risk by making healthy changes to your diet and lifestyle. Smoking, obesity, and a sedentary existence are lifestyle choices that increase your risk of stroke. If you are obese, you most likely also have other risk factors for stroke including high blood pressure, insulin resistance and diabetes, and unhealthy cholesterol levels. By embracing bad habits you hurt your endothelium. You block your arteries. You have a stroke. Your brain dies. You go into a nursing home. You may never come out, or you may lose your independence, forever.

The number one risk of stroke is high blood pressure, which is responsive to exercise.

Hypertension, or high blood pressure, is characterized by a persistent increase in blood pressure, even when a person is at rest. The disorder is one of the most common chronic health problems in the United States, and more than half of all persons over age 60 and older have hypertension.[188] High blood pressure is the biggest risk factor for stroke.[189] If you have uncontrolled high blood pressure, you are seven times more likely to have a stroke than someone with controlled high blood pressure.[190] The risk of ischemic stroke is increased in patients with hypertension, with a linear relationship between elevation of blood pressure and stroke risk even in people who have normal blood pressure. In elderly subjects, systolic blood pressure (SBP) elevation in particular is the most important risk predictor for stroke.[191] Becoming more active can lower your systolic blood pressure by an average of 5 to10 millimeters of mercury (mm Hg).[192]

Hypertension promotes stroke by aggravating atherosclerosis in the aortic arch and cervicocerebral arteries.[193] High blood pressure adds to the workload of the heart and arteries. The heart must pump harder, and the arteries carry blood that is moving under greater pressure. If high blood pressure continues for a long time, the heart and arteries may not work as well as they should. As blood circulates, it exerts pressure on the walls of the arteries. Elevated blood pressure causes endothelial injury, which disrupts the blood-brain barrier, leading to a deposition of plasma proteins and eventually degeneration of the blood vessel. This activates a clotting cascade, leading to thrombosis.[194] When blood vessel walls thicken with increased blood pressure, cholesterol or other fat-like substances may break off of artery walls and block a brain artery.

Having high blood pressure and not getting enough exercise are closely related; small changes in your daily routine can make a big difference. Regular physical activity makes your heart stronger. A stronger heart can pump more blood with less effort. This decreases the force on your arteries, which in turn lowers your blood pressure. This is as elementary as it gets.

Through exercise, you can lower your systolic blood pressure or keep it from rising as you age. But to keep your blood pressure low, you need to keep exercising. It takes about one to three months of regular exercise to have an impact on your blood pressure. You must incorporate exercise into your lifestyle as the benefits last only as long as you continue to exercise. Becoming more active can work better than medications designed to accomplish the same.

Type 2 diabetes increases your risk of stroke and is responsive to exercise.

Multiple studies have shown that people with diabetes are at greater risk for stroke compared to people without diabetes, regardless of the number of health risk factors they have.[195] Overall, the health risk of cardiovascular disease (including stroke) is two-and-a-half times higher in men and women with diabetes compared to people without diabetes. In fact, more than 65 percent of people with diabetes die from heart disease or stroke.[196] Moreover, when people with diabetes have a stroke, they often fare worse than individuals without diabetes; diabetes is associated with an increase in overall stroke mortality.[197]

There are two types of diabetes. Type 1 is an autoimmune disease where the immune system attacks and destroys the insulin-producing beta cells in the pancreas. Type 1 accounts for about 5 to 10 percent of diagnosed diabetes in the United States, and it develops most often in children and young adults. The remaining 90 to 95 percent of people with diabetes in this country have type 2. This form of diabetes is most often associated with older age and obesity. The pancreas is usually producing enough insulin, but for unknown reasons the body cannot use the insulin effectively—a condition called insulin resistance—and after several years, insulin production decreases. The result is the same as for type 1 diabetes: glucose builds up in the blood and the body cannot make efficient use of its main source of fuel.

The excess glucose (blood sugar) or insulin (a hormone that regulates glucose) in the bloodstream can damage the arteries that deliver oxygen to the brain and predispose them to atherosclerosis, which, as discussed, creates blood-flow abnormalities and compromised oxygen supply to the brain.[198] When the oxygen supply is cut off, other arteries can usually deliver oxygen by bypassing the blockage. In people with diabetes, however, many of the bypass arteries are also affected by atherosclerosis, impairing blood flow to the brain.[199]

There is unequivocal and strong evidence that physical exercise can prevent or delay the progression of type 2 diabetes in individuals with compromised glucose tolerance. Also, lifestyle interventions, including diet and physical exercise, can result in a reduction of around 50 percent in diabetes incidence that persists even after the individual lifestyle counseling has stopped. In addition, short–term randomized studies have confirmed that physical training based on endurance and/or resistance exercises can improve blood glucose control in type 2 diabetics.[200] It therefore goes without saying that physical exercise is an important factor in warding off type 2 diabetes and managing the disease. But, I'll say it anyway.

Here is how it works: when you exercise, your muscles need extra energy or fuel (e.g., glucose). When you experience short bursts of exercise like walking up the stairs or a quick sprint to remove your toddler from harm's way, the muscles and the liver can release stores of glucose for fuel. However, when you set out to engage in a moderate exercise regime, your muscles take up glucose at almost 20 times the normal rate, and this lowers blood sugar levels. Be careful and try not to overdo it with intense exercise, as it can have the opposite effect and actually increase your blood glucose levels. When you intensely exercise, this is perceived as a stress on your body; the stress hormones that tell your body to increase available blood sugar to fuel your muscles are released. This does not mean that if you are a diabetic you should refrain from really working it, you may just need a little insulin after an intense session. Of course, as with any exercise routine, you should check with your doctor and perhaps even a nutritionist.

The American Diabetes Association recommends 150 minutes of moderate to vigorous physical activity each week, including aerobic exercise and weight training. According to its report, this physical activity is associated with greater cardiovascular risk reduction. This is consistent with a number of studies.[201] The report states that in the absence of contraindications, people with type 2 diabetes should be encouraged to perform resistance exercise three times a week, targeting all major muscle groups.[202]

If you have type 2 diabetes or are on the path to that disease process, I hope that I have encouraged you to make a lifestyle change that incorporates long-term resistance training and aerobic exercise into your daily routine. Of course, an experienced trainer should supervise any exercise program initially and a pre-exercise medical assessment should be performed as appropriate. If you have diabetes, you must understand when it is safe to exercise.

There is an association between a history of hypertension and type 2 diabetes, giving you a joint reason to exercise.

As I previously noted, hypertension and type 2 diabetes are independently linked to increased risk of stroke incidence and stroke-related mortality. A recent study looked at the combined effects of hypertension and type 2 diabetes on the incidence of stroke and stroke mortality. The researchers found that both are greatly increased in patients with both conditions. They opined that because hypertension and type 2 diabetes often occur concomitantly, it is possible that a large proportion of stroke cases thought to be related to hypertension might also be attributable to unrecognized type 2 diabetes.[203] If exercise and diet can help prevent the processes of both diseases, and both diseases are leading causes of disability (which will lead to your lack of independence), are you still reticent to climb onto the treadmill or take that walk around the block?

Stroke Prevention and Diet

Eating a healthy diet is probably the most effective way to keep a low stroke risk, because it can protect you from developing high blood pressure, diabetes, high cholesterol, obesity, and more. Eating healthy does not mean eating a whole bag of baked chips because you would otherwise eat their unhealthy counterpart. Likewise, it does not mean that you are entitled to eat a couple of doughnuts because you only ate a salad without dressing for lunch. I myself have employed that faulty logic and have, at times, found myself resting upon a big butt because of it. And that is precisely why I have coined the phrase "buffatt" to describe what I look like after a jaunt to Vegas that involves seeking sustenance from its omnipresent eating stations. But what does "eating healthy" really mean? Here are four quick tips you can go by to ensure healthy eating.

1. Eat small portions. Eating more than your body requires forces your metabolism to store the extra calories and increases your body weight.

2. Eat salt in moderation. Salt makes the body retain fluid, which in turn increases your blood pressure. Try to eliminate sources of excessive salt from your diet, such as canned foods or soy sauce.

3. Make unhealthy meals the exception, not the rule. Keep your urges for fried foods and other delicious, but not-so-healthy dishes under control, and maintain a healthy diet otherwise. Make fast food, if you crave it, only an occasional splurge.

4. If you drink, do so in moderation. It has been suggested that wine may actually help reduce stroke risk. But don't reach for that bottle just yet. While studies hint that one to two glasses of wine per day may be helpful in reducing risk, further studies are needed. Like anything else, alcohol should be consumed in moderation.[204]

As people age, their cholesterol levels rise. Before menopause, women have lower total cholesterol levels than men of the same age. After the onset of menopause, women's low-density lipoprotein (LDL) cholesterol levels tend to rise.[205] High levels of LDLs, the "bad" cholesterol, may increase your risk of atherosclerosis. In excess, LDLs and other materials build up on the lining of artery walls, where they may harden into plaque. High levels of triglycerides, a blood fat, also may increase your risk of atherosclerosis. In contrast, high levels of high-density lipoprotein (HDL) cholesterol, the "good" cholesterol, reduce your risk of atherosclerosis by escorting cholesterol out of your body through your liver.[206]

Elderly people often suffer from a deficiency of vitamins B_6 and B_{12} and folic acid.[207] In fact, vitamin B_{12} deficiency is estimated to affect 10–15 percent of people over the age of 60.[208] Vitamin B_{12} is produced by bacteria and is found exclusively in animal products: liver, meats, eggs, dairy products and fish. There is virtually none in foods of vegetable origin.[209] It is also produced by the bacteria in the large intestines but this is not absorbed into our bodies. To be absorbed, the vitamin first has to be released from food by the action of pepsin and acid from the stomach. It then binds with a protein produced by the stomach called intrinsic factor. The complex passes through the intestines to the last twelve inches of the ileum, just before the commencement of the large bowel, where it is finally absorbed.[210] Only a limited amount, up to two micrograms, can be absorbed after any one meal. It is absorbed into the blood stream and stored in the liver.

In the elderly there is often a decrease in either the output of acid or intrinsic factor by the stomach and this will reduce the absorption of vitamin B_{12} even from an adequate diet.[211] Abnormally high blood levels of the amino acid homocysteine, which occur with deficiencies of vitamins B_6 and B_{12} and folic acid have been linked to an increased risk of coronary artery disease and stroke.[212] Some experts believe that homocysteine is a major risk factor for stroke, second only to high blood pressure.[213] Homocysteine appears to be toxic to the cells lining the arteries and to contribute to blood clotting. Specifically, abnormal homo-cysteine levels can contribute to atherosclerosis in at least three ways: (1) a direct toxic effect that damages the cells lining the inside of the arteries; (2) interference with clotting factors; and (3) oxidation of low-density lipoproteins (LDL).[214] In light of the fore-going, you should discuss with a medical professional how to incorporate vitamins B_6 and B_{12} and folic acid into your diet.

Alzheimer's Disease and Exercise

Some people will develop Alzheimer's disease due to a combi-nation of genetics and environmental factors. It is an age-related disease. It is not a given that you will get it after you reach 85, but you are at a 50 percent risk if have you have other suscepti-bility factors. You cannot change your genetics or your age, but you can certainly influence your environment and lifestyle, which may act as a trigger for the timing of the onset. Although it is never too late to begin, the most important time for adjusting your health and lifestyle is at middle age because that is when the plaques that are so devastating to brain function begin to form.

No one knows how the Alzheimer's disease process begins. The etiology of the disease is multifactorial. According to the National Institute on Aging, during the preclinical stage of Alzheimer's disease, people are free of symptoms but toxic changes are taking place in the brain. Abnormal deposits of proteins form amyloid plaques and tau tangles throughout the brain, and once-healthy neurons begin to work less efficiently. Over time, neurons lose their ability to function and communicate with each other, and eventually they die.[215] Before long, the damage spreads to a nearby structure in the brain called the hippocampus, which is essential in forming memories. As more neurons die, affected brain regions begin to shrink. By the final stage of Alzheimer's, damage is widespread, and brain tissue has shrunk significantly.

There is recent evidence of the role of vascular risk factors in the onset and progression of Alzheimer's disease. Many people with early dementia or Alzheimer's disease symptoms may have actually experienced small strokes that damaged the brain's neurotransmitters. By keeping cholesterol levels in check, the arteries are free and clear of plaque that can cause stroke. Many scientists espouse a vascular theory, while others point to insulin resistance—two chronic conditions that contribute to stroke as well. In fact, according to a study done by Columbia University Medical Center researchers, a history of diabetes and elevated levels of cholesterol, especially LDL cholesterol, are associated with faster cognitive decline in patients with Alzheimer's disease. These results add further evidence of the role of vascular risk factors in the onset and progression of the disease.[216]

Those who suffer from high blood pressure, strokes, and diabetes are typically overweight, suffer stress, smoke, have clogged arteries, **and do not exercise.** When you do exercise, you maintain good blood flow to the brain, and thereby protect against heart attack, stroke, and diabetes—risk factors for Alzheimer's and other dementias. You also encourage new brain cells to proliferate. Unless we affirmatively do something to inspire new neurons, they will be forever lost. This process of creating new neurons and connections is called neuroplasticity. This term encompasses a process that results in the brain reorganizing itself and creating *new* neural pathways and connections through mental and physical exercise.

Studies have shown that active laboratory animals have more hippocampal memory cells than inactive animals, and that cardiovascular fitness is associated with greater parietal, temporal and frontal cortical tissue.[217] I have seen these mice in action. It is startling to see how much more efficient the fit mouse is on performance measures than its lazy rodent cronies. Additionally, a report prepared for the National Institutes of Health states that exercise can stimulate the production of growth factors, which are molecules produced by the body to repair and maintain nerves.

If these reasons aren't enough for you to be motivated to get physically fit, let me add this: Exercise also reduces stress levels, and people with stressful lives are around two to three times more likely to develop Alzheimer's disease than others. It is now widely accepted that cortisol, a hormone that is produced in the adrenal gland in response to times of stress, plays a central role in the development of Alzheimer's disease. In the short term, this hormone can be helpful. Following a stressful experience, cortisol levels rapidly increase in the blood stream, improving short-term memory formation and adapting the body's physiology to deal with the situation effectively. But long-term stress leads to prolonged elevated levels of cortisol within the blood stream, which contribute to the development of Alzheimer's disease.[218]

In a study with genetically modified mice, University of California, Irvine researchers found that when young animals were injected for just seven days with dexamethasone, a glucocorticoid similar to the body's stress hormones, the levels of the protein beta-amyloid in the brain increased by 60 percent. This is significant because when beta-amyloid production increases and these protein fragments aggregate, they form plaques—one of the two hallmark brain lesions of Alzheimer's disease. The scientists found that the levels of another protein, tau, also increased. Tau accumulation eventually leads to the formation of tangles, the other signature lesion of Alzheimer's.[219] They concluded that, in humans, increases in circulating cortisol could increase the pathology present in the brain, and thus could make people develop Alzheimer's disease faster.[220]

Virtually any form of exercise, from aerobics to weightlifting, can act as a stress reliever. If you're not an athlete—even if you're downright out of shape—you can still make a little exercise go a long way toward stress management. For the greatest overall health benefits, experts recommend that you do 20 to 30 minutes of aerobic activity three or more times each week, and some type of muscle strengthening activity and stretching at least twice each week. However, if you are unable to do this level of activity, you can gain substantial health benefits by accumulating 30 minutes or more of moderate-intensity physical activity each day, at least five times a week.

If you have been inactive for a while, you may want to start with less strenuous activities such as walking or swimming at a comfortable pace. Beginning at a slow pace will allow you to become physically fit without straining your body. Once you are in better shape, you can gradually do more strenuous activity. Talk to your doctor first. But then, whatever it takes, just do it. Please. You will be honoring your wish to remain independent.

Alzheimer's Disease and Diet

Some studies suggest that higher dietary intake of antioxidants, vitamins B_6 and B_{12}, folate, unsaturated fatty acids, fish, and Omega 3 fatty acids are related to a lower risk of Alzheimer's disease, but reports are inconsistent. Likewise, modest to moderate alcohol intake, particularly wine, may be related to a lower risk of developing Alzheimer's. The Mediterranean diet (which is not really a diet but rather a way of eating) may also lower your risk. The "diet" includes a reliance on vegetables, fruits, beans, whole grains, nuts, olives, and olive oil, as well as cheese, yogurt, fish, poultry, eggs, and wine. These foods—which are whole foods, not processed with any ingredient list longer than my legs—provide thousands of micronutrients, antioxidants, vitamins, minerals, and fiber that work together to protect against chronic disease.

Rush University Medical Center researchers conducted an informal survey of 6,000 people initially unaffected by Alzheimer's disease on Chicago's South Side. They gathered a staggering amount of data about this group's dietary habits and then regularly evaluated a subgroup for signs of Alzheimer's disease. They found that foods rich in vitamin E—such as oil-based salad dressings, fortified cereals, green leafy vegetables, cantaloupe, seeds, and nuts—were associated with a reduced risk of developing the disease. They also found that people who ate fish at least once a week were 60 percent less likely to develop Alzheimer's disease than those who rarely or never ate fish. They think that the key ingredient is the n-3 polyunsaturated fatty acids in fish. From these data, the team made an association between high intakes of saturated and trans-unsaturated fats and Alzheimer's disease.

What does all this mean? It means it's better to limit fatty meats, full-fat dairy products like butter and milk, and vegetable shortening. Since research indicates that oxidation of the brain over time causes mental deterioration, the researchers speculate that vitamin E, as an antioxidant, may combat that process. The n-3 fatty acids found in fish share chemical similarities to substances found in the brain's gray matter. These substances help transmit signals to the brain, allowing for learning and memory storage. As for the "bad fats," these culprits are associated with high cholesterol, and (as you already know) high cholesterol has been shown to be bad for both the heart and the brain.[221]

Interestingly, randomized clinical trials of supplements of vitamins E, B_{12}, and B_6, and folate, have shown no cognitive benefit, and randomized trials for other nutrients or diets in Alzheimer's disease are not available. In other words, the existing evidence does not support the recommendation of specific supplements, foods, or diets for the prevention of Alzheimer's disease.[222] Obviously, however, since being overweight can cause diseases that make you more susceptible to getting Alzheimer's disease, moderating your food intake would still be wise.

The constant thread in my research is that lifestyle choices—not drugs—are the key to successfully keeping this insidious disease at bay. There are no drugs to keep a person from getting Alzheimer's disease; there are only drugs that make the symptoms more manageable, and only for a time. Ultimately, preventing cell loss is more effective than trying to repair a damaged brain. The goal is to keep your brain healthy, just like we try to keep our hearts and blood pressure levels healthy. This is not just about eating right and exercising; it is also about avoiding depression and toxic substances like cigarettes. (If you are over 65 years old and smoke, your chances for developing Alzheimer's increase by over 70 percent.) It is about getting enough sleep and exercise. It is about staying engaged.

Fall Prevention and Exercise

Among older people living in the community, falls are a strong predictor of placement in skilled nursing facilities; interventions that prevent falls may therefore delay or reduce the frequency of nursing home admissions.[223] Falls account for 25 percent of all hospital admissions, and 40 percent of all nursing home admissions. Of those individuals admitted to nursing homes, 40 percent do not return to independent living and 25 percent die within a year.[224] The most effective way to prevent fall injuries such as hip fractures is to combine exercise with other fall prevention strategies.[225]

The ability to perform daily activities and maintain independence requires strong muscles, balance, and endurance. Balance plays an important role in everyday activities such as walking, getting up out of a chair, or leaning over to pick up a grandchild. Balance problems can reduce your independence by interfering with activities of daily living. Guidance from the National Institute for Clinical Excellence (NICE) on the assessment and prevention of falls in older people includes evidence to show that Tai Chi taught in 15-week courses can improve muscle strength and balance in older people, thereby reducing the risk of falls. Indeed, Tai Chi is an excellent means of balance and coordination training. It can decrease blood pressure, lessen the velocity of sway, increase stability and balance, reduce the fear of falling, and increase confidence in balance and movement.[226]

Strength training improves muscular endurance and strength, range of motion, and flexibility. It can be done using free weights, weight machines, or resistance bands. Walking also improves balance, ankle strength, walking speed, and falls efficacy, while also decreasing falls and the fear of falling.[227] If you suffer from arthritis or other joint conditions, try water aerobics; it is gentle on joints and provides the same benefits that other "land exercises" provide.

One last word about falls. Many of my clients fall because they are on too many medications or on medications with contraindications. They are on these medications because they have chronic illnesses that must be managed. But if you stay fit, eat right, control your stress and manage your weight, you will not have chronic health issues and will not need pharmaceuticals. Don't let a fall be your demise.

There is not much any of us can do to change the fact that age is a risk factor for chronic illness. We can, however, make lifestyle choices that promote normal blood pressure and thwart diabetes. If you make good choices now, you can lessen your chances of stroke and Alzheimer's disease—tragedies that do not have to be an inevitable fact of aging. I have said all that I can say on this subject and all I have left is a plea for you to treat your body well by choosing whole foods and exercising every day.

CHAPTER 10

A Little Psychobabble Never Hurt Anyone

The connection between the mind and body has been the topic of many a news show, magazine article, and research study. Yet, how our mental state impacts the quality of our lives as we age—specifically in our later years—is still, from my experience as a gerontologist, underestimated. There is a broad range of mental health problems in later life; mostly, there is a lot depression. In fact, the highest suicide rates of any age group are among persons aged 65 years and older. There is a widespread belief that these problems are a natural part of the aging process, but this is not the case. It is important to remember that most people remain in good mental health throughout their lives. Many people do not understand the relationship between a healthy mind and body; without good mental health, the quality of our lives is compromised. Because depression is not a normal part of aging, good mental health can be a choice.

Choose to be prepared for the things that you can control. Be the master of your well being.

My perception is that much of the depression in older adults can be attributed to loss and isolation, the feeling that they are alone and have lost friends and perhaps even a spouse. I have been witness to many losses and reactions thereto. But because I have not perfected the most effective way to conquer loss, whether in the form of a loved one's death, the loss of a sense or capability, the loss of beauty and vitality, or the loss of a driver's license, I would be seriously over stepping my boundaries in providing home grown advice on how to overcome *your* losses.

What follows is a culmination of my research over the years and the resulting theories that I have crafted about overcoming grief. I too strive to accomplish what I write about. I speak in terms of loss because at the core of our existence as humans we reach an apex where youth and maturity converge and we find ourselves wondering where that went. When we acknowledge that it will not return, we may spend precious time and resources trying to re-capture and rein-vigorate what we have lost. If this were not the case, there would not be a multi-billion dollar industry dedicated to this proposition. Ultimately, if we are lucky, we come to understand that it is the rela-tionships we have forged that cushion the blow of these losses. For me, it is the loss of those relationships through death or incapacity that serve as motivation to understand how to conquer grief.

On a personal note, I will admit that even when I am surrounded by my children and husband, I feel alone. Even when I am in front of a big crowd, all eyes locked onto my mouth, awaiting an answer to a struggling person's problem, I feel alone. In recognizing this about myself, I also recognize why many people speak of God in a way that I do not. They do not feel alone. So, when I feel this way, I try to move myself toward a spiritual center, always coming back to the notion that we come into this life alone and that our death is the same way. I may feel alone, but I have no expectations that others are here to fill a space that can make me feel empty. In other words, I have spent time thinking about *why* I feel the way I do and *how* I can move myself through it. I hope my words will encourage you to do the same, and to find ways to look out for yourself and the people around you.

This chapter provides an overview of some common mental health problems in later life, including those associated with loss. It should be a useful resource for you, as well as your family members, caregivers and friends. The basic premise is that a good plan, based on solid information, will mitigate many of the fears and insecurities that foster emotional instability as we age.

Of course, mental health problems that are chemical in nature or somehow physiologically induced can affect each of us at any time in our lives. Many older people who have mental health problems may not be diagnosed or get treatment. The early detection and treatment of mental health problems can lead to significant improvements in the quality of not just an older adult's life, but all of our lives. It is imperative to speak to your doctor if you experience the symptoms of depression that I describe in this chapter.

And, if you think that you have to move to the next chapter because this does not apply to you, or because you just don't have a taste for psychobabble, try and refrain. It is so important to understand how depression impacts our ability to age successfully. I define this as **being able to hold onto your dreams and aspirations and God given independence.** If this freedom from institutional bondage is not compelling enough, you should know that scientists all agree that depression is not good for your brain function. In fact, studies have indicated that depression may as much as double your risk of developing dementia, including Alzheimer's disease.[228] Everyone, you included, wants to avoid this.

A study published in the April 2008 issue of *Archives of General Psychiatry* showed a correlation between depression and

Alzheimer's disease. While not conclusive, it did cause the researchers to think that depression may change brain chemistry in such a way that the brain becomes more susceptible to Alzheimer's disease. A second study, in a 2008 issue of *Neurology*, investigated whether a history of depression was associated with the later development of Alzheimer's disease. The researchers found that people who have had depression are almost 2.5 times more likely to develop Alzheimer's than those who haven't had depression. Those who experienced depression before the age of 60 were almost four times more likely to develop Alzheimer's disease. Both studies cautioned about making assumptions about a direct link, but the mere suggestion of a relationship is enough to give me pause.[229]

I will do anything I can to ward off this iniquitous disease. I try to be happy every day, even when I am faced with what can seem to be daily defeat. I try to enjoy the infinitely short time we get to be on this planet. I was not always this way. I was depressed for years. I woke up every morning with the Beatles lyrics to "A Day in the Life" in my head: "got up, fell out of bed, dragged a comb across my head…." That is a sad, weird, depressing song. I had nothing to be sad about, but I was lost.

I had stopped working for seven years to raise my kids and felt like I could never get a job again or be of value in the workforce. I was chemically a mess from going into menopause at 40. My daughter got sick and my mother, with whom I had a very tumultuous relationship, got sick with cancer and died. I even took a shot at being a professional poker player (for about two weeks!), but the universe did not reward that, and even losing a dollar made me feel bad about myself. It took some seriously hard work, counseling, good friends, and a great husband to pull me out of that slump. I realized that the gift of life was worth fighting for and a happy life was my battle. In the introduction, I told you that I was a fighter and I fought my way out of my depression. Now I sing "Good Day Sunshine" when I wake up—to me there is no longer a choice. Striving to be happy when I wake up is as mandatory as brushing my teeth.

To reiterate, nearly half of all nursing home residents have Alzheimer's disease or a related disorder; it is why they are there. In the previous chapter, we discussed how maintaining a healthy body impacts the onset and progression of Alzheimer's disease. Now you know that maintaining a happy disposition and positive attitude can also help stave off the disease. Please do not say that you do not need to adjust your attitude or seek assistance while also admitting that you are terrified of getting this insidious disease. This cognitive dissonance will not serve you. Here is your chance to be well and independent.

Identifying Depression

I am a pragmatist. I understand that many elderly adults face significant life changes, including a great deal of loss and other stressors that put them at risk for depression. Those at the highest risk include older adults with a personal or family history of depression, failing health, substance abuse problems, or inadequate social support. As I will describe below, prescription medications can also trigger or exacerbate depression, as can chronic or severe pain, cognitive decline, or one's body image due to surgery or disease.

Sometimes, we just feel fed up, miserable, or sad. Sometimes there is a reason, but sometimes these feelings just come out of the blue. These feelings generally don't last for more than a few days and they don't stop us from getting on with our lives. However, you may be experiencing depression if you have any of the following symptoms and they last for more than two weeks and interfere with your everyday life:

- Feelings of sadness or hopelessness
- Difficulties with daily activities
- Difficulties concentrating
- Changes in your sleep pattern
- Changes in your eating pattern

Never assume that a loss of mental sharpness is just a normal sign of old age. It could be a sign of depression or dementia, both of which are common in the elderly. Since depression and dementia share many similar symptoms, including memory problems, sluggish speech and movements, and low motivation, it can be difficult to tell the two apart. In fact, doctors have been known to misclassify depression and dementia based on ageist notions of older adults. There are, however, some differences that can help you distinguish between the two:

Someone with depression...	**Someone with dementia...**
• Has relatively rapid mental decline	• Experiences slow mental decline
• Knows the correct time, date, and place; can name other people	• May be confused and disoriented, or become lost in familiar locations
• Has difficulty concentrating, may have memory lapses that can worsen mood	• Has consistent trouble storing new information (e.g., may not remember what, if anything, was eaten for dinner)
• Has slow but normal language and motor skills	
• Notices or worries about memory problems	• Has impaired writing, speaking, and motor skills; may have difficulty naming common objects like a pen, lamp, or birthday cake
	• Doesn't notice memory problems or seem to care

Before being diagnosed with depression, elderly adults should be screened for common health issues that can also affect mood. These include:

- Hormonal imbalances
- Thyroid problems
- Vitamin B_{12} deficiency
- Other nutritional deficiencies
- Electrolyte imbalances or dehydration

Illness and Depression

When undergoing evaluation for depression, long-term or severe health issues should also be taken into account. Chronic medical conditions, particularly those that are painful, disabling, or life-threatening, can understandably lead to depression. Illnesses that affect the brain can also cause depression through the disease process itself. Medical conditions that commonly trigger depression include:

- Heart attack or disease
- Parkinson's disease
- Stroke
- Alzheimer's disease
- Multiple sclerosis
- Cancer
- Diabetes

Medication-Induced Depression

Some medications can actually cause symptoms of depression or make a pre-existing depression worse. All medications have side effects, but harmful drug interactions or a failure to take a medication as prescribed can also contribute to depression. The risk of medication-induced depression is particularly high for elderly individuals with multiple prescriptions. Some medications that can induce depression include:

- Steroids
- Painkillers
- Hormones
- Arthritis medication
- High blood pressure drugs
- Heart disease medication
- Tranquilizers
- Cancer drugs

Bring a list of all medications to the doctor so that he or she can help you determine if any of the prescriptions are the cause of depression symptoms you may have.

What Can Trigger Depression?

Older age can be a time of dramatic upheaval that tests physical, psychological, and spiritual boundaries. We experience many adjustments and these can be very stressful, especially if we don't feel prepared or supported. Some of the more obvious changes are retirement, loss of a spouse, death of friends, loss of physical function and good health, and loss of independence (a multi-faceted concept). Being on a fixed income may cause uncertainty about your ability to be cared for. Contacts with friends and acquaintances may have been curtailed and your own health may be declining. Some things may be gender specific. For example, men often lose their ability to have or maintain an erection. Women experience a loss of girlish sexuality and may feel that their physical beauty has faded. Some people adapt well to change and embrace it with a sense of wonderment. Others fear the unknown. In whatever camp you reside, if you feel at all vulnerable, weakened by illness, or overwhelmed by an ever-increasing sense of mortality, the process is usually more difficult.

I hope I have convinced you that being depressed is something you need to avoid if you want to stay independent. But how can you be proactive in this endeavor? If you live long enough, so many things can create an opportunity for depression. The first step is to accept that knowledge is power. Please benefit from my interviews with dozens (and dozens) of older adults who candidly discussed the triggers of their depression. These triggers seem universal. If you can anticipate them, you can make a plan to combat them.[230]

Retirement

In 1883, Chancellor Otto Von Bismarck of Germany had a problem. Marxists were threatening to take control of Europe. Fearing that his countrymen would succumb to their ideology, he proclaimed that he would pay a pension to any nonworking German over age 65. This was a brilliant yet empty gesture, since the average lifespan during the late 1800s was 50 years old. Bismarck not only undermined the Marxists, but also set the arbitrary world standard for the exact year at which old age begins. In short, he planted the seed for our modern day notion of retirement.

Despite the fact that when someone should retire is a capricious line drawn by a paranoid official, the impact of retirement should not be underestimated. For many, work is central to their lives and provides structure to their days, a sense of purpose, and many times a social network. While retirement may be anticipated, it is common for individuals to experience mixed feelings about leaving an environment so integral to their daily existence. Anxiety about what the future will hold is common. Feelings range from being hurt and angry to wondering how retirement will affect their relationships to worrying if they will have enough money to live on. People find that they have a lot more free time when they retire and, as a result, relationships with partners and children often change, requiring an adjustment for both the retiree and family. Many older people feel more successful when they become more active and develop a regular structure to their days.

If you are on the precipice of retiring, now is a good time to reflect upon the activities that you longed to participate in when you were busy raising your children or working 40–60 hours a week. Did you always want to bike, draw, write, teach, be more civically engaged? Think about what you want the picture of your life to look like and paint it in advance. Talk about it. Dare to dream about your future as filled with fun and joy and then wait for that day with the anticipation of a child at the counter of a candy store.

Many people worry about the financial challenges that retirement may bring. This is why having a plan is so essential. By doing a little advance planning a person can exert control over this variable. Living in limbo is very difficult for most people, and when you add the vulnerability that many older people experience, it can make it all the more difficult. Don't be a victim of circumstance because *you are not a victim*. You may not be as physically powerful as you once were, but you still have power through action.

If you are worried about whether you have enough money to pay for long-term care, if you don't want to be a burden to your children, if you don't want to go into a nursing home—get long-term care insurance. This product can enable you to save your hard-earned money and get care at home or in a dignified setting. Instead of spending your entire life's savings on skilled nursing care, you can pass it on to your heirs. You cannot depend on the government to take care of you.

If you are worried about being able to survive on a fixed income, and if you are over 62 years of age and have a home, look into a reverse mortgage. Why sweat the small stuff? Why worry that you will run out of money to pay for food and medication?

Why wonder if you can make home improvements because you have limited resources? You can finance your needs with an asset for which you have worked your entire life. Let that asset work for you now. (I will explore long-term care insurance, reverse mortgages, and a host of other financing tips in more detail in the next chapter.)

As you look toward retirement, take advantage of planning seminars. Helen Dennis, Ph.D., author of *Project Renewment*, notes that whatever your plans, spouses or partners should be encouraged to attend retirement planning and education programs together. If you are married, you should both have equal access to information and discussions. Facilitators and instructors can design nonthreatening exercises to determine the extent to which spouses and partners are financially literate and have similar or divergent thoughts about use of time, relocation, and other subjects. Develop your communication so that you can establish a good relationship in retirement and so that you will have the tools to accomplish your goals.

According to Dennis, as boomer women begin to retire, they are likely to be equal participants in retirement education and decision making.[232] By the same token, nonworking spouses or partners of both genders must play an integral role in the planning process; their job descriptions may be more demanding and diverse than those of any paid employee. All couples should have equal access to useful retirement information and enlightening discussions that lead to secure, meaningful, healthy, and joyous futures.

Bereavement

With a long life come friends, family, maybe even a partner. But a long life also brings loss, and the loss of a spouse or partner can be one of the most harrowing and stressful events we endure. If you have not learned this about me yet, my husband is my world. He is my best friend (though if you asked me yesterday, I may have said otherwise!). When I hear someone speak of the loss of her spouse, the pain cuts though my heart; because I am a professional I must keep my tears, with my eyes wobbling in their sockets. This type of loss is painful at any time in our lives, but when you grow older you may be less able to cope and move on. The intensity of emotion can be magnified by a confluence of events that happen at this stage in life.

Mutual dependence for love and support is a cornerstone of a long marriage. For many couples who have weathered the storms of a long relationship, a spouse is more than someone married long ago—there is great friendship and everlasting respect for one another. A spouse is a best friend, a guide, and a companion. When half of a partnership is suddenly gone, the will to survive is often shattered.

When your spouse dies your universe changes. You are in mourning—feeling grief and sorrow at the loss. Feelings of numbness, shock, and fear are natural. You may feel guilty for being the one who is still alive. If your spouse dies in a nursing home, you may wish that you had been able to care for him or her at home. At some point, you may even feel angry at your spouse for leaving you. All of these feelings are normal. There are no rules about how you should feel. There is no right or wrong way to mourn.

According to an oft-cited Finnish study, recently widowed men and women experience a heightened death rate in the months after their spouses die. That study, which involved a large cohort of individuals, found that the greatest hike in mortality comes in the first seven days. The most common cause of death during the critical post-death week is heart attack, possibly brought on by the stress of the spouse's death and exacerbated by an inability to sleep in the first days of grief.[233]

If you have recently lost your spouse, it is critical that you have help coping with the immediate aftereffects. It is vitally important to recognize that you may be struggling and to know what can help you through it. When we grieve, we feel both physical and emotional pain. People who are grieving:

- Can have trouble sleeping.
- Often cry easily.
- Show little interest in food.
- Experience problems with concentration.
- Have a hard time making decisions.

Many of these stages of grief are unavoidable. But there are things you can do to take your mind off the pain. For example:

- Take a walk with a friend or meet with old friends.
- Go to the library to check out books.
- Volunteer at a local school as a tutor or playground aide.
- Join a community exercise class or a senior swim group.
- Be part of a chorus.
- Sign up for bingo or bridge at a nearby recreation center.
- Join a bowling league or a sewing group.
- Offer to watch your grandchildren or a neighbor's child.
- Consider adopting a pet.
- Think about a part-time job.
- Try to eat right, exercise, and get enough sleep. Avoid bad habits such as drinking too much alcohol or smoking, which can put your health at risk. Take care of your body; grief can be hard on your health.
- Be sure to take your prescribed medications. Remember to see the doctor for your usual visits.

As you adjust to your new normal, it is so important that you tend to your own mental health. Draw on all of the resources available to you to help you heal:

- Don't think you have to handle your grief alone. Sometimes short-term talk therapy can help. Professionals such as mental health specialists, clergy, and doctors can all be of assistance.
- Grief and loss support groups are also extremely helpful. The opportunity to process and share feelings with others experiencing similar difficulties can be invaluable in the healing process. Check with hospitals, religious groups, and local government agencies to find out about support groups.
- Let family provide nurturance and support. At the same time, don't rely on your children to pave the way for you during this transition. Most children will be supportive, but will be proud and grateful if you allow them to lead their lives while you begin to reconstruct yours. They are grieving too. It will take time for the whole family to adjust to life without your spouse.
- Try not to make any major changes right away. It's a good idea to wait for a while before making big decisions like moving or changing jobs.

The grieving process, *as long as its length is not too extreme*, is one of the most vital components of the healing process. For some people, however, mourning can go on so long that it becomes unhealthy. If you're having trouble taking care of your everyday activities, like getting dressed or fixing meals, this can be a sign of serious depression and anxiety.

My mother-in-law recently passed away. She existed on this planet for 12 years after my father-in-law's death, but she did not live. She was only 62 when he passed. Her light went out when her best friend died; her funny, charming, and witty disposition was lost. It seemed like nothing could resurrect this. She tried, but all who knew her as the wife of Judge Magistrate Ralph Geffen knew that she was half a person. From that day forward she abused herself with smoking and alcohol and pain relievers. She traveled (which was her second love) but her tales were muted by a monotonous cadence. This is not what her husband would have wanted and it was very painful for her children to witness.

Although a grieving person may experience a number of depressive symptoms such as frequent crying and profound sadness, grief is a natural and healthy response to bereavement and other major losses. There is a difference, however, between a normal grief reaction and one that is disabling or unrelenting. While there is no set timetable for grieving, if it doesn't let up over time or extinguishes all signs of joy—laughing at a good joke, brightening in response to a hug, appreciating a beautiful sunset— it may be depression. If your sadness stays with you and keeps you from carrying on with your day-to-day life, talk to your doctor or a mental health professional.

When you feel stronger, there are some financial and legal things that you may need to think about:

- Writing a new will.
- Looking into a durable power of attorney for legal matters and a power of attorney for health care in case you are unable to make your own medical decisions.
- Putting any joint assets (such as a house or car) in your name.
- Checking on your health insurance as well as your current life, car, and homeowner's insurance to make sure that you have adequate coverage or coverage at all.
- Signing up for Medicare by your 65th birthday.

- Paying state and federal taxes if, due to your grief, you failed to do so.

When the time is right, and only when the time is right, go through your spouse's clothes and other personal items. It may be hard to give away these belongings. If it is too hard to part with everything at once, do it in incremental steps. For example, instead of parting with everything at once, you might make three piles: one to keep, one to give away, and one "not sure." Ask your children to help. Think about setting aside items to give to your children or grandchildren as personal reminders of your spouse.

If you are lonely or feeling isolated, don't shy away from technology. I can empathize with those who feel that learning how to operate newfangled devices is too complicated. One of my clients did not want to get a computer and try email because she thought it would be another avenue for thieves. As with anything else, you have to be vigilant, but I do not believe that on balance her fear was a good justification for refusing to try her hand at the Internet. There are not only limitless learning opportunities through chat rooms that focus on innumerable subjects, but computers and other devices are great ways to stay connected with family members who live far away. You can even reconnect with lost friends. There are devices and programs that enable you to see the person you are speaking with in real time, and vice versa. I believe that technology can change a lonely person's life. If you can manage to learn how to use the Internet and a smartphone, I guarantee you that you will open yourself up to a world that will astonish you.

Moving From Your Home

Seniors are typically attached to their homes because they symbolize stability and comfort. Even in the face of compelling reasons to find better living arrangements, most seniors would probably go to extra lengths just to remain "home." (That is why I devoted an entire chapter to the topic!) Unfortunately, however, it is not always an option.

Whether an older adult is involuntarily forced to change his or her residence or chooses to do so independently, it can be very stressful. In fact, research shows that the elderly population is extremely susceptible to what is known as Relocation Stress Syndrome (RSS). This condition, also known as transfer trauma, was recognized as an official nursing diagnosis in 1992. It is characterized by a combination of physiologic and psychological disturbances such as anxiety, confusion, hopelessness, and loneliness, all of which can significantly affect behavior, mood, morbidity and even mortality. Studies show that 31 percent of seniors decrease their social networks when they move, and they have a 30 percent possibility of hospitalization within a month of doing so. RSS can last for several months, often persisting a year or longer. In fact, in one study, more than half of the older adults who were interviewed did not feel at home in long-term care after residing there between two and seven years.

Symptoms of RSS can include exhaustion, sleep disturbance, anxiety, financial strain, grief and loss, depression, and disorientation. In older people, these symptoms can quickly become exacerbated by dementia, mild cognitive impairment, poor physical health, frailty, lack of support system, and sensory impairment. The most reliable study done on RSS found that the problem is better handled and accepted when a psychological and sociological approach to treatment is taken, rather than a medical approach, which invariably means the use of medication. Thankfully, if you know the potential effects of a move before you undertake it, you have a better chance at avoiding these problems.

So what can you do if you must move from your home?

If you are faced with the need to move from your home, there are many options available and I have explored these in-depth in earlier chapters. Read through the information, seek advice, and choose the best option for you. Fear of the unknown can make moving from home into care more difficult. There are many things that can be done to make the process easier:

- Be involved in the decision-making as much as possible.
- Visit the place where you will be living before you move.
- Meet the other residents and become familiar with the staff and environment.
- Make a plan for your move.
- Find a moving company that caters to seniors. These companies usually have senior relocation specialists to help coordinate all aspects of the process.
- Make a list of who you should contact to tell them about your move, including the post office, utility services, your friends, and neighbors. Don't forget to give them your new address and phone number.

It is normal to feel anxious, stressed, or angry at the time of a move. Even if you are prepared, you may panic. It takes time to settle into any environment and after you have had time to catch your breath, it should get easier. Surround yourself with your belongings, photos of family, or favorite books. Maintain contact with your family and friends. Remember to tell people how you are feeling at this time.

How can you help a loved one transition to a new home?

If you are reading this book as a caregiver, it is important to know that there are also things that you can do to make your loved one's move less stressful. For example:

- Discuss the move in detail, use pictures or, if possible, take them on a tour of the facility they are going to. Reassure them continually and keep them in the loop.
- Whenever possible, allow them to make decisions. Let them feel some control, even if this is only possible in small amounts (such as in the choice of which pictures or blankets to take along).
- Be patient and recognize that they may require extra attention and reassurance after the move.
- Stress the positive aspects of moving such as socialization, freedom from the demands of maintaining a home, and increased opportunities for both mental and physical activity.
- Make sure that the new surroundings incorporate the past and that there are photographs and nick nacks in place as reminders that only the structure has changed, not the people or the history.

In some cases, it may make sense for your parent to move into your home. In some instances there could be real benefits to this. If your parent is healthy and able-bodied, is personally close to you, and gets along with everyone in your family, the benefits could be enormous. He could be very helpful around the house and with your children, while the activity and socialization can help him stay engaged. It could be a great time for him to bond more with your kids and he could be another positive adult role model for them to learn from.

But, there are other circumstances where it might not work out as well. The first item I would assess is whether your parent is physically able to take care of himself. Does he need round the clock attention? Does he have any physical conditions that you might not be able to handle in an emergency? Can he be left alone if you have to run out for a few hours? These things are important to consider because chances are your life is pretty full and stressed as it is now. Having to be responsible for another person's safety and well-being is not only a full time job, but a very stressful one at that. It can become very difficult if you have to make arrangements every time you need to leave the house.

Next, you have to consider family dynamics. Be realistic and ask yourself if your current relationship with your parent is conducive to him moving in. Does your parent get along with the rest of the family? If you, your spouse, or child has had personality clashes with this parent in the past, do not believe those issues will suddenly disappear when he moves in. In fact, it will be just the opposite, because you will all be spending that much more time together. Even if you personally get along with each other, be sure to take your spouse and children into consideration. If you have a parent that drives your kids or spouse crazy, you can end up alienating your own family. The new stress level in your house will make everyone unhappy.

If you are the one contemplating a move to live with your grown children, you should consider everything I have already mentioned, but there are also other issues for you to take into account. For example, you may want to consider whether they will cramp your style. It is no mystery that we get set in our ways. Although you may love your children and grandchildren dearly, you may not end up liking them very much when you are with them 24/7. This may be why grandparents who are happy to see their grandchildren are often even happier when the rugrats go back to their own homes where they can terrorize others. It can be a wonderful opportunity to spend time with the people who love you must, but be realistic about your own limits and the limits of your family.

Like all stages of life, older age brings its own challenges, but with the support of family, friends, and the many organizations ready to listen and help, these challenges can be overcome.

Loss of Intimacy

It is frequently assumed that elderly persons lose their sexual desires or that they are physically unable to perform. The media often portray the elderly as sexually undesirable, and the whole notion of older adults having sexual relations is somehow perverse. This is especially true for women who tend to outlive their male counterparts by seven or more years and who are left without sexual partners in the later years. Society has condoned the relationships of older men and younger women, but tends to ostracize older women who establish relationships with younger men. Elderly women are the neuters of our culture.

Society has not left older men unscathed by its portrayal of their sexual capacity. With so much attention paid to Viagra, it is assumed that older men are unable to become aroused or maintain a state of arousal, a notion that is at odds with human sexuality and is degrading to men. Impotence is not exclusively a biological phenomenon. There can be a number of factors involved, such as boredom, fatigue, overeating, excessive drinking or medications, and medical or psychiatric disabilities. Nevertheless, elderly men are often seen as impotent buffoons, which unnecessarily fuels fear about loss of sexual prowess. Societal jokes about elderly men and sex—such as the bumper sticker: "I'm not a dirty old man, I'm a sexy senior citizen"—do nothing but ridicule them.

While both men and women can continue to have satisfying sex lives as they grow older, and while many seniors continue to enjoy their sexuality into their eighties and beyond, it would be irresponsible to refrain from mentioning some challenges that older adults could face.

In both sexes, hormone levels decline with age and changes in desire and sexual function are common. Health can also impact your sex life and sexual performance. If you or your partner is in poor health or has a chronic health condition such as heart disease or arthritis, sex and intimacy become more challenging. Moreover, certain surgeries and many medications—including blood pressure medications, antihistamines, antidepressants, and acid-blocking drugs—can affect sexual function.

As an older adult you are entitled to your sexuality. In fact, it is good for your mental health and self-esteem. It is perfectly acceptable for you to have sexual feelings and for couples to have sexual feelings about each other and to act on them. Even if your desire and ability to have intercourse have declined, the need for touch and intimacy continues. Without intimacy, any adult, regardless of age, can get despondent and depressed. Adapt to your changing body and know your limitations. Focus on ways of being sexual and intimate that work for you and your partner. Here are some ways to facilitate this adaptation:

- **Communicate with your partner.** Open discussion of sex has become more common in recent years, but many older adults come from a generation where it remains a taboo subject. But openly talking about your needs, desires, and concerns with your partner can bring you closer and help you both enjoy sex and intimacy more.

- **Talk to your doctor.** Talking about sexual issues with your doctor can help you maintain a healthy sex life as you age. Your doctor can help you manage chronic conditions and medications that affect your sex life. Some older men have trouble maintaining erections or reaching orgasm. Your doctor may be able to prescribe medications or other treatments for these problems.

- **Expand your definition of sex.** Intercourse is only one way to have fulfilling sex. Touching, kissing and other intimate sexual contact can be just as rewarding for both you and your partner. Realize that as you age, it's normal for you and your partner to have different sexual abilities and needs. Be open to finding new ways to enjoy sexual contact and intimacy.

- **Change your routine.** Simple changes can improve your sex life. Change the time of day when you have sex to a time when you have the most energy. Try the morning—when you're refreshed from a good night's sleep—rather than at the end of a long day. Because it might take longer for you or your partner to become aroused, take more time to set the stage for romance with a romantic dinner or an evening of dancing. Try a new sexual position or explore other new ways of connecting romantically and sexually.

- **Seek a partner if you're single.** It's never too late for romance. It can be difficult starting a relationship following the loss of a partner or after being single for a long time, but socializing is well worth the effort for many single seniors. No one outgrows the need for emotional closeness and intimate love. If you start an intimate relationship with a new partner, be sure to practice safe sex. Many older adults are unaware that they are still at risk of sexually transmitted diseases, including AIDS.

- **Stay healthy.** Staying healthy can help your sexual performance. Keeping up your health by eating regular nutritious meals, staying active, not drinking too much alcohol, and not smoking or using illicit drugs are all important to your overall health. Follow your doctor's instructions for taking medications and managing any chronic health conditions.

- **Stay positive.** The changes that come with aging—from health problems to changes in appearance and sexual performance—leave many men and women feeling less attractive or like they're less capable of enjoying or giving sexual pleasure. Discussing your feelings with your partner can help. Feeling angry, unhappy, or depressed will have a strong negative impact on your sex life. Professional counseling or other treatment can improve your sex life—and your well-being.

For more information on sex and aging you can visit to the following websites:

The AARP/Modern Maturity Survey:
http://www.aarp.org/relationships/love-sex/info-1999/aresearch-import-726.html

American Association of Sex Educators, Counselors, and Therapists (AASECT):
http://www.aasect.org

Age Page: Sexuality in Later Life (National Institute on Aging):
http://www.nia.nih.gov/health/publication/sexuality-later-life

Sleep Deprivation
Sleep deprivation leads to poorer quality of life and, in the elderly, it can lead to a number of more specific problems. Older

adults who have poor nighttime sleep are more likely to experience depression, as well as attention and memory problems, excessive daytime sleepiness, more nighttime falls (a leading cause of injury and death among seniors), and use of more over-the-counter or prescription sleep aids.

While it is true that seniors sleep less deeply and wake up more often throughout the night (which may be why they also sometimes nap more often during the daytime), it is a myth that older people don't need as much sleep as the average person. In fact, adults require about the same amount of sleep from their twenties into old age. Yet, insomnia is more common for seniors. Older adults sleep less and wake up more often during the night for a variety of reasons:

- Increased sensitivity to changes in their environment, such as noise.
- Anxiety and the concerns of aging.
- Lower levels of melatonin, the hormone that promotes sleep.
- Frequent urination.
- Pain from arthritis.
- Sleep apnea.
- Restless Leg Syndrome.
- Medications.

If you're having trouble sleeping, try these techniques for getting more shut-eye:

- **Get set.** Wake up at the same hour every day; too much time in bed can lead to restless sleep. Exercise and eat meals at set times to help get sleep back on track.
- **Get sun.** No matter your age, daylight is extremely important because it helps regulate the sleep/wake cycle. Spend as much time as possible outdoors or near sunlight.

- **Get checked.** Medication can interrupt sleep. A doctor can recommend adjusting the timing or dose of specific medications, or possibly switching to alternative prescriptions.

- **Eat Smart.** Avoid alcohol, caffeine, and spicy or sugary foods four to six hours before bedtime. These all contain substances that will keep you awake.

- **Exercise regularly,** especially in the late afternoon or early evening, because it raises your body temperature above normal a few hours before bed, allowing it to start falling just as you're getting ready for bed. This decrease in body temperature can be a trigger that helps ease you into sleep. **You should not** exercise within three hours of your bedtime, as that acts as a stimulant.

- **Avoid sleep interruptions.** Don't sleep with a restless or yippy pet, and close your door to minimize light and noise.

- **Relax before bedtime.** Enjoy a warm bath or light snack (bananas, warm milk, chamomile tea, and oatmeal are good options).

- **Avoid long naps during the day.** Naps can disrupt your sleeping pattern.

- **Avoid trying to sleep.** The more you "try" to sleep, the more difficult it becomes.

- **Use your bed for sleeping.** Reserve your bed for nighttime sleep and the occasional nap, rather than for unrelated activities like reading or watching television.

- **Check your medications.** Medications may increase your sleep difficulties. If you must take any sleep aides, make sure that there are no potential conflicts with other medications you are taking. I once noticed that a client was on both Aricept and Ambien, despite the FDA's warning that Ambien can cause memory loss!

See your doctor if you're not getting restful sleep at night and/or if you are unable to wake up refreshed. The National Institutes of Health (NIH) website includes a sleep and aging section that provides detailed information about the importance of sleep for seniors, some of the sleep difficulties people encounter as they age, and the symptoms and treatment of various sleep disorders, such as insomnia, sleep apnea, and movement disorders. For more information on the relationship of sleep and healthy aging visit the NIH website (www.nih.gov) and type "sleep" in the search box.[234]

Loss of Your Driver's License

All too often I am asked by adult children about "taking away" their parents' driver's licenses. This question and its resolution go to the heart of one's independence. Sometimes it is the tone of the question that leads me to great discomfort. It is as if the adult child is annoyed that his or her parent doesn't just toss over the keys and submit like a puppy. Sometimes, it is a question asked with indignity—like, "doesn't this old person know that the jig is up?" To those who use this tactic, STOP! It is mean and insensitive. Speaking these words is the last resort. Instead, employ empathy.

Last year I met with a family to discuss how to care for their 87-year-old father and husband, a former charismatic public relations guy. He was slipping away slowly, but nonetheless, slipping away. Although the doctor told him that he could no longer drive, he said that he did not hear that. He wore hearing aids in both ears. So, to clarify, I asked him what he meant by the word "hear." Did he literally not hear him or was he going to a happy place when his doctor was speaking those life-altering words?

The next day he got into a fight with a taxi cab driver, found the keys to the car, and drove from Santa Monica to an imaginary appointment in downtown Los Angeles. What was going through his head as he plowed into a one parked car after another? The answer: nothing. There was nothing going through his head. The classical music provided a background to his delusional, life-threatening excursion. All I got from him was the relief he felt at not having a memory of anything, since that "would have been very scary." For him, there was no connection between his conduct and the real possibility that many innocent people could have been killed.

We don't have to worry about him driving again. The LAPD who surrounded him when his vehicle finally came to a halt took away his license and Buck's Towing took away his totaled vehicle forever. He spent the rest of his life calling the DMV <u>every day</u> to get his license back.

Can you imagine not being able to grab the keys and run to the store or out for coffee or to the movies? I know that it is hard to fathom why someone who is a danger to themselves and possibly innocent civilians, maybe a child, wouldn't just cough up the keys, but it is a complicated issue. I have seen families resort to disabling a parent's car, removing the car from the place of residence, confiscating car keys, and canceling auto insurance. In response, their mildly demented parents have responded by calling the police for a supposedly stolen car, having the disabled car towed to a repair shop, and having a locksmith replace keys. Again, this is difficult for everyone.

This is hardly going to be a detached intellectual analysis. My father is teetering on the edge right now and he has rebuffed my recommendation to relinquish the keys. My dad is a tough guy from Chicago. He played football when they had no protective gear. He boasts about the guys whose teeth were knocked out by his blows. He can still beat anybody to the punch on Jeopardy. But at the same time, he is blind in one eye and has a temporary license. The last time I drove with him I told him I was scared he was going to kill me. His response? "I gave you life, I can take it away." He was joking. I was appalled. If the potential of killing me was not persuasive, then I had nothing left in my arsenal.

To those of you who are imminently facing this crossroads, I ask you to consider that your children are not mean. They are correct. How would you feel if you killed someone? What if you ran into a crowd of people at a farmer's market? What if, as the result of an accident, you lost your life's savings and this rendered you and your spouse penniless? How would you pay for your housing and your care? If someone suggests that you relinquish the keys, please consider that they may have a valid point.

If you are faced with having a conversation with someone who may need to give up their keys soon, it is helpful to know that the kind way to get someone to cooperate with anything is through rational and logical negotiation. If you realize that your parent associates having keys with being able to get out of the house and socialize or get chores done or go to meetings, you have to be prepared to provide a legitimate alternative plan. Having a plan will help your parent (or you) live independently, and will prevent isolation and the possible need for long-term care place-ment in a nursing home. It may mitigate depression. In Los Angeles, where convenient public transportation is as plentiful as rain in Texas, how is a person supposed to get from point a to point b without a car? If you can solve that problem, then you can buffer the blow.

I wish that I could provide a pat answer to what type of trans-portation services exist in any given community. There are some common types that may be available for the elderly such as individual door-to-door service, fixed routes with scheduled services, or ridesharing with volunteer drivers. You can call a local senior center or senior services agency to find out what is available in your area. In some communities, a local Area Agency on Aging (AAA) will arrange, monitor, and support programs that provide transportation services for older adults. The National Transit Hotline (800-527-8279) can provide the names of local transit providers that receive federal money to provide transportation to the elderly and people with disabilities.

As far as my father is concerned, at first I was going to recommend that he sell his car and put the money into a special account to be used for cab fare. I even calculated it. He could get everywhere he might want to go (including the racetrack) for $300 a month, so his fund would last him for a good three years. When he turned 85, we could re-evaluate. In the meantime, he could schmooze on his phone and tell the driver what a stupid route he was taking, just like when I drive him around. Then, after doing some research (yes, I put a lot of thought into how to approach him), I realized that there might be a less restrictive option.

In my case—and perhaps in yours as well—the solution is not to take away the keys, but to negotiate some limitations on driving based on the statistics of senior accidents. Seniors are most susceptible to having accidents at intersections in urban areas. Even though they tend to average the fewest miles, the elderly often drive in the most dangerous driving environments: Local roads where frequent intersections and heavier traffic increase the probability of vehicle conflict and accident risk for drivers of any age.[235] The crash is usually caused by the older driver's failure to heed signs and grant the right-of-way. At stop sign-controlled intersections, older drivers may not know when to resume driving.[236] Left-hand turns are the most problematic, and glare sensitivity makes night driving and certain situations like entering and exiting tunnels more difficult. With this knowledge, you can have an intelligent conversation about the parameters of your parent's, your spouse's, or your own driving and not throw the baby out with the bathwater.

Several studies show that older drivers tend to be more adaptive to their limitations when they are aware of what they are; they tend to have a greater tendency toward "self-regulation" than their younger counterparts. Seniors are aware of their changing abilities and adapt their driving habits accordingly, by making shorter trips, totaling fewer miles, and driving much less at night, in heavy traffic, and in bad weather.[237] Empowered by this information, I had a very productive conversation with my dad about the parameters of his driving and the avoidance of some routes.

My dad loves to drive to Las Vegas from Los Angeles. He has taken this route many times. It does not require much maneuvering as it is on the open highway. That is not a problem. He also goes back and forth to the same places and understands the rhythms of the routes. Until such time that he becomes more vision impaired or cognitively disabled, we have agreed to put the topic on the shelf. He went from being very disturbed by and angry about our conversation to hugging me at the end.

If you are lucid but know that you get confused or disoriented when you drive, try to think of the loss of your license in terms of an act of selflessness. To give up the privilege of driving so that you can possibly save the lives of others can be a source of pride and you can avoid the embarrassment of having that privilege formally stripped from you.

This informal analysis is similar to what 28 states and the District of Columbia do when older adults attempt to renew their licenses. Some states impose accelerated renewal cycles with shorter periods between renewals, requirements to renew in person rather than electronically or by mail, and testing that is not routinely required of younger drivers (vision and road tests, for example). If your appearance or demeanor at renewal, a history of crashes or violations, or reports by physicians, police, or others cast a doubt on your continued fitness to drive, state licensing agencies may require you to undergo physical or mental examinations or to retake the standard licensing tests (vision, written, and road) when you seek a renewal.

After reviewing your fitness to drive, the licensing agency may allow you to retain your license, or they may refuse to renew your license, or suspend, revoke, or restrict it. Typical restrictions prohibit nighttime driving, require the vehicle to have additional mirrors, or limit driving to specified places or a certain radius from your home. In states where the renewal cycle is not shorter for older drivers, licensing agencies have the authority to shorten the renewal cycle for individual license holders if their condition warrants it. If you know that you have a problem, you can be the one to control the conditions under which you will stop driving.[238] Feeling empowered rather than feeling like a victim can go a long way in maintaining good mental health.

Last night I visited one of my dear clients. I told her that being happy and positive will help her keep her memory, which sadly she is losing. She replied, "Okay, I will remember that!"

The triggers of mental health decline that I have just shared with you are not meant to be an exhaustive list. I am not a psychologist. Rather, this chapter was borne out of my experience with older adults and the research that I have done in an effort to help them.

If you are worried about a mental health problem ***please seek help***. Sorting out whom to talk to and where to get help can be very confusing. Sometimes just talking to a friend helps. Confide in someone you trust. The best place to start is often with your own doctor, who can then refer you to the most appropriate service. Bring a family member or friend with you if it makes you feel more comfortable. Whatever you do, don't be afraid to talk about how you are feeling and to ask for help. While being diagnosed with a mental illness or depression can be frightening, many people say that putting a name to the symptoms can be comforting. Knowing what you are experiencing is the first step to recovery.

If you have thoughts of suicide, please call a suicide hotline or crisis support organization.

The National Suicide Prevention Lifeline is a suicide prevention telephone hotline funded by the U.S. government. They provide free, 24-hour assistance. 1–800–273–TALK (8255).

The National Hopeline Network has a toll-free telephone number offering 24-hour suicide crisis support. 1–800–SUICIDE (784–2433).

CHAPTER 11

Getting Old Is an Expensive Habit

Those who are 80 and older and who have already lived out their retirement years by traveling and volunteering are now facing another, unanticipated phase—old, old age. The growth rate of this population segment is twice that of those 65 and older and almost four times that of the total population. In the United States, this group now represents 10 percent of the older population and will **more than triple** from 5.7 million in 2010 to over 19 million by 2050. The most common question that I have to resolve for my old, old clients is whether they are going to outlive their money. This comes from people who never thought they would live as long as they have lived.

The average cost of long-term care in the United States can run between $40,000 and $80,000 a year, depending on the level of care one needs and the setting in which the care is provided. These figures vary by state, but then again so does the cost of living.[239] If you have Alzheimer's disease, the cost of care can be even higher. According to a 2010 MetLife Mature Market Study, 68 percent of assisted living communities surveyed nationwide provide dementia and Alzheimer's care for their residents. The study also found that the national average for Alzheimer's care costs at assisted living communities is $4,762 per month, or $57,144 annually. Where a community specializes in Alzheimer's care *only*, the cost of care tends to be $1,000–$1,500 higher per month.

According to the 2011 MetLife Long-Term Care IQ Survey, 60–70 percent of 65-year-olds will require long-term care services at some point in their lives.[240] The IQ Survey was conducted to determine how it is that so many Americans between the ages of 40 and 70 know what long-term care is and what it may cost, but most continue to be unaware of their potential need for long-term care or how they will pay for it. Over four in 10 people who participated in the survey (43 percent) were able to correctly identify the national average monthly cost for assisted living, yet two-thirds (66 percent) were unable to identify which programs or insurance policies would pay for long-term care services. What is your long-term care IQ?

It should not escape mention that according to a study by the AARP Public Policy Institute, between 1991 and 2007 the rate of personal bankruptcy filings among those ages 65 or older jumped by 150 percent; the most startling rise occurred among those ages 75 to 84, whose rate soared, increasing by 433 percent.[241] And if you think that you can finance your existence with credit cards, think again. Two-thirds of Americans who filed for bankruptcy did so because of credit card debt.[242] Besides having more credit card debt compared to younger bankruptcy filers, 45 percent of those aged 65 and older also had more plastic in their wallets. According to a University of Michigan study, 67 percent of people age 65 and older who filed for bankruptcy in 2007 cited credit card interest and fees as a culprit, compared with 53 percent of those under 65. When one considers that these bankruptcy figures reflect trends before the recession began in 2008, it's fair to assume the situation has worsened in the past few years due to job losses and diminished retirement portfolios and housing equity.

Using credit cards when you do not have the resources to pay the bills—or, in the case of older adults, the time to recover financially from a financial hiccup—may reduce some stress in the short term, but it is non-productive in alleviating the actual problem in the long term. Many seniors fall back on this maladaptive coping mechanism and find themselves in a quagmire that sets them back both physically and emotionally. In my experience, when my clients have their backs up against the wall with increasing financial pressure, their self-assessments decline and they experience a diminishing ability to care for themselves.

I don't know about you, but on any given day there are usually only two out of my four children who like me. So unless your child is rich, benevolent, *and* still likes you, you'd better beef up (or should I say pork up?) your piggy bank, as the cost to self-insure can be astronomical. This chapter provides practical advice on how to finance long-term care by discarding dated notions of retirement, and by using private sector and government resources such as those available through the Social Security Administration, the Veterans Administration, Medicaid, and community-based programs that currently exist to help offset, if not completely pay for, long-term care.

Let's get to it!

Work

The financial meltdown left many on the precipice of retirement in a tailspin. At least one in four older Americans is either postponing his retirement or seeking to return to the workforce, while four in 10 employers have designed programs to encourage late-career workers to stay past traditional retirement age. Do you take umbrage at the notion that you may have to work for the man for another five years? Even the ninety-one-year-old former U.S. Supreme Court Justice John Paul Stevens thinks he may have "jumped the gun" on retirement and that it would "... perhaps be appropriate to increase the retirement age under the Social Security law."

I don't even know what the word retirement means. It has no relevance to my universe. As with many notions we have, somewhere along the line we have been snookered into believing that retirement is an inevitable phase. The indoctrination starts when we are born. We are expected to develop in a certain manner and within a certain time frame. Our public school system treats us like widgets, labeling "square pegs" as outliers. We are moved like sheep from grade to grade with the expectation that college, marriage, family, buying a home (and taking on huge debt), retirement, and death naturally follow in order. Just like that and then...poof, it is over.

Who can forget the hero pilot, Chesley B. "Sully" Sullenberger III, who landed a packed passenger plane on the Hudson River after Canadian geese disabled the engines? This 58-year-old man not only made a miraculous emergency landing but was reported to walk the aisles twice to make sure that every passenger had been rescued. At 58, he was two years from mandatory retirement for commercial pilots.

Despite the stepwise abolishment of mandatory retirement through the federal Age Discrimination in Employment Act in the 1960s and 1970s, mandatory retirement age rules still prevail in some private- and public-sector occupations including: state and local police (ages 55–60) and firefighters (ages 55–60); federal firefighters (age 57); federal law enforcement and corrections officers (age 57); air traffic controllers (age 56, if hired after 1972); and commercial airline pilots (age 60). Mandatory retirement age restrictions were introduced in these occupations several decades ago, primarily for ensuring safe and effective conduct, but I believe they are outdated. Even as far back as 1978, research has asserted that the fears regarding older workers are not based in fact. According to a Harvard Business Review study, the performance of older workers and their work attitudes far exceed the younger cohort's.[243] Overall, the majority of human resource professionals recognize that the advantages of hiring older workers outweigh the disadvantages.[244]

I think we should strike the term retirement from our vocabulary and treat each day as part of a continuum of how we feel and what we believe and what we need at any given moment. Maybe one day I will want or need to slow down. Maybe I will *need* to continue to work and will not want someone taking on ageist notions of whether I am right for a position. Who knows? Just because I cannot fathom exiting the workforce when I reach a certain date, that does not mean that I won't. If you asked me 15 years ago if I would ever consider plastic surgery I would have definitely said no. I was pretty back then and I wore no make-up. Now, as I stare in the mirror, pulling on my face and contorting it until it is taught, I am leaving that option open.

For those of you who can relate to this, there is good news. In a study titled *After the Recovery*, Barry Bluestone and Mark Melnik from the Dukakis Center for Urban and Regional Policy at Northeastern University estimate that by 2018 there could be more than 5 million unfilled jobs in the United States. Why? Because the number of baby boomers leaving the workforce will exceed the supply of new workers coming from younger generations. According to their research, because these people have already begun to exit, it is easy to calculate what the workforce will look like. Between 2008 and 2018, the 65–74 age group will grow by nearly 44 percent and the 55–64 group will grow by nearly 40 percent. By contrast, the pool of people aged 45–54 will drop by 8 percent and there will be a 4 percent decline in the number of persons aged 35–44. In short, there is an impending worker shortage that will need to be filled by us boomers.[245]

Social Security (Is that an oxymoron or what?)

Have you ever wondered what would happen if you took your Social Security benefits now, before you hit 66? This friends, is really not a black and white decision. Social Security is not a simple system. You will have to employ a calculator, or your fingers. You might even feel like you need to have a degree in math with an emphasis in actuarial science. I will try to simplify this for you because, if you are cash strapped, you may have to look at dipping into this pseudo savings repository. The cost of making the wrong (and actually complex) decision can be huge.

Please know that regardless of when you take Social Security and when you stop working, you **must** enroll in Medicare when you first become eligible at 65, or you could face financial penalties in the form of higher premiums. For those of you who are about to turn 65, you can start the process in advance, which is what I recommend. Plan, plan, plan…and then let go and have fun!

Here is a general overview. You can start collecting Social Security anytime from age 62 to 70. The later you start, the bigger your monthly benefit, depending on when you were born. If you were born from 1943 to 1954, you will receive your full (normal) benefit when you hit 66. If you cash in at 62 you will get 25 percent less than your normal benefit. If you wait until you are 70 you will get 32 percent more than your normal benefit. If you were born after 1954 you will have a slightly higher "normal" retirement age, which means you will take a somewhat bigger hit for claiming your benefits early and get somewhat less of a bonus for waiting until you reach 70.

If you claim early while you are still working, you will receive an earnings penalty. Until you reach the full retirement age, for each $2 you earn above $14,640 in a given year, you lose $1 of your annual Social Security benefits. If you can wait until after 66, benefits don't get cut no matter how much you earn. If you reach 66 this year, you can earn $38,880 in salary in the months before you reach 66, without affecting your benefits. And for each $3 you earn above those ceilings, you will lose $1 in benefits.[246]

Still with me? Here is how it works in real terms. Let's say that you are turning 62 this June and you currently earn $50,000 a year. You could collect about $988 a month once you reach 62 years. If you wait until you are 66, you will get $1,391 a month. If you wait until you are 70, you will receive $1,934 a month. Here is the tricky part: These benefit amounts are not as dramatically different as they might sound. **If you live long enough, you will end up taking the same *total amount* of benefits no matter when you claim.** But gender matters here. If you are a woman, you are expected to live longer, and that means you are more likely to reach the age at which waiting to collect a bigger check pays off (and no, simply dressing like one won't work!). If you are of the male persuasion, you may want to raid your security earlier.

If you don't need an early check to make ends meet, and particularly if you're single, this could be a significant factor in your decision. You can check out the calculator on the Social Security website that will give your average life expectancy without regard to your health or family history. There are a lot of Internet sites that will calculate your life expectancy by taking into account your health, family history, exercise, eating, drinking and driving habits and even social relationships. Any of these calculations should be taken with a grain of salt, of course. But the bottom line is that if you're in poor health, and you want to get some of your tax dollars back, it can make sense to claim Social Security as early as possible.

Personally, I would not take benefits while I was earning a decent salary. Some think of waiting to take benefits as insurance against outliving their money. It is like buying a larger, inflation-adjusted lifetime annuity for a lot less than you could buy a commercial annuity, even from a low-cost, no-commission provider. (Then again, I am a woman! Hear me roar!)

The real brain twister arises in the context of married couples. Put simply, they are treated better. If one partner dies, the survivor can claim the deceased spouse's check instead of his or her own, assuming the deceased spouse's check is bigger. In the actuarial and insurance businesses, this is known as joint mortality. Where there are two individuals, there is a greater chance that at least one of them will live a long life and collect a bigger check. This means that the higher earning spouse should delay benefits well past 66, to buy that higher lifetime "second-to-die" annuity that will benefit the other spouse.

While both you and your spouse are alive, you are entitled to what you yourself have earned, or up to half of your living spouse's full retirement benefit—whichever is higher. But if you are the low earning spouse and you rely on spousal benefits, you will take an even bigger early claiming hit than a primary wage earner would. For example, if you claim benefits at 62, you will receive only 35 percent of your spouse's full retirement age check, instead of 50 percent. And, you will get no extra benefit for waiting *past* full retirement age to claim your check. So, for example, in a one-income household where the husband is four years older, the couple would receive the maximum benefit if the husband claimed at 70 or if the wife put in for her spousal benefits at 66.

Consider another angle. Let's assume that you and your spouse want at least some cash coming in from Social Security before one of you reaches the age of 70. Once the older of the two of you reaches full retirement age of 66, benefits can be claimed (thereby initiating the process) and then immediately suspended. The spouse can continue to wait for a bigger benefit, while the other spouse is now eligible to claim spousal benefits.

Lastly, once you reach full retirement age, you can choose to take benefits as a spouse, while deferring your own earned benefit until later. So in a two-income marriage where the partners are the same age, one might claim benefits at 66. The other could then claim 50 percent of those benefits as a spouse, while allowing his or her earned benefit to build until 70. Again, this is a way to "purchase" longevity insurance for both of you.

The website of the U.S. Social Security Administration (www.ssa.gov) has a wealth of information on all of these topics. It may seem daunting and confusing at first, but gaining a clear understanding of all of your options will help you maximize your Social Security earnings.

Long-Term Care Insurance

Long-term care insurance is the missing piece in a realistic retirement portfolio. It can be an affordable alternative to using your savings to pay for care, whether that care is delivered to you at home or in a facility. Unlike health care insurance or Medicare, which pay for immediate medical expenses like a doctor's bill, long-term care insurance covers basic daily needs over an extended period of time. Long-term care insurance helps if you can no longer be independent as a result of an accident, illness, or old age.

The government tried to establish a program for long-term care through the CLASS (Community Living Assistance Services and

Supports) Act, which was signed into law by President Obama on March 23, 2010 as part of more comprehensive health care reform. It was designed to provide a cash benefit ($50–$75 per day) to people needing long-term care services. Workers would have to pay into the program for at least five years before they could receive any benefits. Anyone, regardless of degree of disability, could participate, provided they were employed at the time of enroll- ment (and for at least three years during those initial five years). Furthermore, the law required that no taxpayer money could be used to fund benefits. Unfortunately, on October 14, 2011, the Obama administration terminated further work on CLASS. It was determined that the program could not sustain itself for at least 75 years because the premiums were not high enough to fully fund the program. The lack of underwriting caused the risk to be too high. In other words, there was no way to keep it solvent.

It should not surprise you by now to hear that I am a huge proponent of long-term care insurance. My husband and I each have a policy. I got mine when I was 47 because I know that long- term care isn't just something that I *might* need in the distant future. About 40 percent of people needing long-term care are adults ages 18–64. They may have had an accident, a stroke, developed multiple sclerosis, or some other illness. I do not want to bankrupt my family or put my spouse in financial jeopardy should I get sick or become disabled.

We bought our policies after I attended a lecture at the University of Southern California titled, *The Many Faces of Dementia*. At one session there was a panel of three individuals in the beginning to middle phases of the disease. Each was accompa- nied by a caregiver. One woman was 40 years old, and her caregiver was her sister-in-law whose husband also had early onset Alzheimer's disease. There was another brother who had Alzheimer's disease as well. Because each sibling had a 50 percent chance of getting this disease, they all bought long-term care insurance. This woman was not able to say much, but what she did say was that her husband and three children would have been financially devastated had they not purchased the product.

Premiums can vary dramatically depending upon factors such as your age, your marital or partnership status, the level of inflation-adjustment protection you select, the daily benefit, and the benefit period (the length of time your long-term care insurance will pay benefits). In 2012, the annual cost for a policy for a 55-year-old in good health with a three-year benefit period, a 90-day deductible, and 5 percent compound inflation protection was $2,269.[247] Importantly, rate books are changing in 2012; it is doubtful that this price will be truly reflective of 2012 once the year comes and goes, but it can still serve to give you a general sense of the cost of this product.

Unfortunately, insurance companies are discontinuing unlimited lifetime benefits. Therefore, look for a "restoration of benefits" feature that allows the full benefit period to be restored if you recover and you do not use any benefits for a particular period of time. For example, if you have a policy without this benefit that has a six-year benefit period and you have a one-year nursing home stay, you would be left with five years on your policy. With this benefit, if you do not draw on any of your long-term care benefits for two years (or less, depending on the policy) following your stay, the insurance company would be required to restore your original full benefit period. Bear in mind that the average nursing home stay is just under three years. As such, you should probably choose a benefit period of at least four years.

Another alternative is to purchase a benefit increase rider, although this may be illusory in certain situations, especially in policies with a low maximum benefit. For example, if a policy has a $50,000 maximum benefit and the rider increases the daily benefit without increasing the maximum benefit (which is frequently the case), you would reach the policy maximum benefit very quickly. In that situation, the benefit increase rider may not provide a meaningful benefit. It may be more valuable in "duration" policies—those that do not cap the maximum benefit by a specific dollar amount. If you have a five-year policy with no maximum dollar benefit, an increased daily amount of benefits may be more valuable.

These policies can be confusing, mostly because the terms and features vary widely, from when benefits start, to the maximum daily payout, to how long the benefits last and what services are covered. It is imperative that you understand the details of what you are buying. Here is what I recommend you ask when looking for a policy:

1. Is there inflation protection? Getting inflation protection is a great opportunity to hedge against hikes in health care costs. This is a very important feature, and there are various options to choose from; what you purchase is very much dependent on your age.

- If you are under 70, I suggest 5 percent compound inflation. With this option, your daily benefit (and your pool of money) will double every 14½ years. This is the most expensive premium option, but you will be paying pennies on the dollar when you use the policy.

- If you are 70 years old or more, 5 percent simple inflation is usually adequate. This option increases your daily benefit by 5 percent of the original daily benefit each year. For example, a $200 daily benefit will grow by $10 each year.

- Future purchase option (FPO)—also called guaranteed purchase option (GPO)—gives you the option every three years to increase your daily benefit the equivalent of 5 percent compound, but each time at a higher premium. This premium is calculated based on your new attained age and the current rate book. I don't recommend this option because your premiums keep getting higher during retirement when your income is generally reduced, and you can't know what the increase will be until they make the offer.

• There are also other options, such as 3 percent compound and five percent compound that cap after 20 years, as well as some whose increases are tied to the Consumer Price Index.

2. What does the policy cover? Long-term care insurance typically covers out-of-pocket expenses that come with home care, assisted living, and nursing homes. You want to look for a comprehensive policy that allows you to use 100 percent of your benefits anywhere you choose to receive care—whether that is at home, in an assisted living or board and care facility, a nursing home, an adult day care or hospice. The majority of policies are what's called "reimbursement," because they pay the monthly bills you send in, up to your current daily benefit. There are a couple of companies that also offer indemnity policies at higher premiums. With this type of policy, you receive monthly checks (without sending in bills), up to your allowed benefit, no matter how much your actual bills were that month.

Home Care covers your personal care (ADLs), homemaker services and various therapies. The best policies allow you the choice between caregivers who are either certified and hired through an agency and those who are non-family, independent and non–certified, such as friends or through recommendations. An 85-year-old retired teacher client of mine was refused benefits because they did not approve of a caregiver that they had paid for when her husband was ill, claiming that she was "not certified." Get the policy that gives you choice.

Most policies also have an equipment and home modification allowance for things such as grab bars, wheelchair ramps, or chair lifts. That means you can pay for home modifications from your benefit account instead of from your savings.

Facility Care covers your room, board, and care in a nursing home, assisted living facility or board and care facility.

3. Is there a waiting period? These are typically called elimination periods and they are the time that must pass before benefits kick in. A 90-day elimination period, for example, would carry a far lower premium than a policy that starts paying out as soon as you're eligible. However, you must understand that with this type of policy you may have to pay tens of thousands of dollars out of your own pocket for your care until the policy can be used, and this would require a cost benefit analysis of the net savings across the anticipated life of the policy. Many policies waive the elimination period if care is started in the home. Be sure to ask whether the elimination period applies to each stay, or if you need to satisfy it only once. If you have to go in and out of a nursing home or other long-term care facility several times, you want a policy that requires you to satisfy the elimination period only once.

4. We are married. Do we get a discount? Married couples (or those living together in a committed relationship, including same-sex relationships) who purchase long-term care insurance from the same company can often get a 20 to 40 percent discount on their premiums. If you are married, you can also purchase a shared policy. With these policies, the total amount of coverage is pooled between the two spouses. In other words, only one policy (or benefit pool) is purchased from the provider, and both individuals can draw upon it (either simultaneously or separately) when care is needed. If one person dies without having used up all his policy benefits, the survivor gets those unused benefits added to the remaining policy. But keep in mind the possibility that you'll end up needing more care than you originally purchased. In the event that you and your spouse become ill or injured at the same time, the insurance may simply not provide enough benefits to cover such significant expenses. While it would provide some benefits, it can still leave your family without enough readily available resources at their disposal.

5. What if I accidentally let my policy lapse? Policies are guaranteed renewable as long as you pay your premiums. I have seen some clients' policies lapse because they were mismanaging their bills or because they had cognitive impairment. Modern policies require you to designate another individual to get a copy of the lapse notices so that you do not lose your coverage. If you can demonstrate that a lapse was attributable to dementia, there is a five-month grace period to reinstate.

You can also purchase a return of premium benefit, which will ensure that you do not lose your benefits if you let your policy lapse and that, if you do not use your long-term care benefits, your premiums will be returned to your heirs. It is a very expensive rider, however. Some people like this benefit because they feel that it protects them from "wasting" their money. I don't recommend it, however, because it would just take a few months of care to make your return of premium rider null and void.

6. Who approves my claim? When you need access to your benefits, you want a policy that allows <u>your</u> doctor to certify that you need help with two of the six activities of daily living (bathing, feeding, dressing, transferring—moving into or out of a bed, chair, or wheelchair—continence, and using the toilet) or that you have cognitive impairment. The insurance company will also require a care coordinator from an independent company to assess your claim. This individual will also help you develop your Plan of Care and can help you find caregivers and other support services. This benefit is generally included in your policy and is paid for by the insurance company.

7. Is the company viable? It goes without saying that before weighing the pros and cons of different policies, the soundness of the companies selling them should be determined. A. M. Best, Moody's, and other such firms show ratings of insurance carriers, so you can quickly weed out questionable companies. These ratings should be taken with a grain of salt, however, as some insurance companies have many divisions and frequently the grading is misapplied by both the interpreter and the agency. The state insurance office can tell you how long a carrier has been licensed to sell long-term care policies and whether the company has hit existing policyholders with premium increases.

Recently, well-respected and long-entrenched companies such as Unum Group have dropped out of the group long-term care business; Prudential Financial has ceased offering individual and long-term care insurance coverage through employer-based groups. Other notable exits include the Guardian Life Insurance Company of America early last year, MetLife in late 2010, and Allianz Life Insurance Company of North America in 2009. Even if your insurer does pull out, you will not lose your coverage. These companies have set aside reserves for *each* policy and, invested properly, they should grow to cover the claim. If the reserves go below government requirements, the Department of Insurance can step in and try to help get the accounts in order, perhaps by improving the company's financial status. If the Department cannot accomplish this, the assets and accounts will get passed to other similar companies based on market share in order to honor claims. There is also a life and health insurance guarantee association like the FDIC that provides a safety net for each state's policyholders, ensuring that they continue to receive coverage even if their insurers are declared insolvent. For more information, you can visit www.NOLHGA.com.

8. I have heard that companies are not paying claims. Prior to 1988, there weren't any consumer protection laws that covered long-term care insurance policies. (Now there are many.) Also, there wasn't the range of long-term care models and options that now exist. As a result, many older adults who bought these original policies are now having trouble with their claims. Early policies would typically not pay benefits unless the long-term care came followed by (usually within seven to 30 days) a stay of at least three days in a hospital or a skilled nursing facility. In reality, most people don't need long-term care because they are recovering from an acute incident. Rather, they are frail and have chronic illnesses, dementia, or Alzheimer's, none of which require initial hospitalization or skilled nursing facility care. As a practical matter, this prior hospitalization requirement meant that the policyholders received no benefits. Now most but not all states have outlawed these exclusions. Make sure that any policy you consider does not have this provision. IT IS NOT WORTH IT.

A company may try to deny a claim based on a self-serving and anachronistic reading of the definition of the type of care you desire. For example, they may question whether the assistance you need with your activities of daily living is "stand by" (excluded by old policies) or "hands on," or they may have hidden exclusions. Even nowadays, you have to be very careful to understand how the proposed policy defines "care at home" or "eligible provider." Does this include assisted living or board and care? Does it require the provider to be licensed in a manner that is not supported by your state's laws? Or does it in reality only allow nursing home coverage? Try to get a policy that has an alternative plan of care provision. This will give you flexibility in deciding where you will receive care. It removes the opportunity for ambiguity about where you can have services delivered. The bottom line is that you must pay careful attention to policy conditions that make it difficult to qualify for benefits and coverage exclusions.

One of the objections you may have to purchasing this type of policy is that it acquires no cash value. If the premiums increase and you just can't afford it anymore, you may lose all of the money that you have already poured into it. It will simply be gone. It is true that you might pay your premiums for years, get hit with rate hikes you can't afford, and then face the tough decision of whether to drop your policy—losing any chance of collecting benefits—or try to struggle on, paying the higher rates. In this case, you could lower your daily benefit slightly or take fewer years of coverage to lower your premium.

If that still was not affordable, you could take advantage of the contingent non-forfeiture benefit that many companies offer. This benefit allows you to use the premiums you have already paid as a future benefit without paying any more. If your contract does does not have this provision and you have paid $2,000 a year for 15 years (or $30,000 total), it could be very disconcerting if you have to give it up. But, if you don't drop the policy and you do subsequently need it, you could be looking at hundreds of thousands of dollars you can use for your care. This is precisely why I recommend that you choose a policy with a premium that you think you can live with—now and into retirement.

The possibility of losing the premium investment causes many people to come up with long-term care savings plans of their own. They think that they will just put $3,500 a year away and self-insure. This has theoretical appeal, but in reality it is not sound. Take, for example, someone who has purchased a long-term care policy ($200 per day; four-year benefit period; 5 percent compound inflation) for a $3,500 annual premium. In 25 years, she would have paid $87,500 in premiums but would have a long-term benefit of $942,000. If she had instead invested the $3,500 each year (and not many are disciplined enough to do this), and earned a consistent rate of 5 percent interest (which is difficult to do these days) her savings would have grown to $167,000, which would only cover about eight months of care. I think you can see why I don't recommend this strategy.

You might also be thinking, *What if I never use the insurance? I will have wasted so much money on premiums.* It is hard to overcome the mindset that unused long-term care insurance is wasted money. But seriously, we never wake up and say, *Darn, I didn't get to use my flood insurance today.* We do not want to use our long-term care insurance, yet if we live long enough, we are likely to do just that. I do not worry about the fact that there is no cash surrender value, I worry that I will be able to afford to stay in my home or somewhere more dignified than a nursing home if I get sick.

When I speak of the benefits of long-term care insurance, I also find myself having to counter the objection that a policy typically only covers three years of care and that many people live long beyond that cap. What happens when your illness or disability lasts beyond the coverage you purchased? In a worst-case scenario, a person in nursing care might outlive by many years the coverage that he purchased, wiping out his savings. If you are especially concerned about this, you might consider a partnership policy, developed by private insurers and state governments. These plans let you qualify for Medicaid's long-term care benefits while you still have a good amount of savings to spend on other things or to leave to your family.

Normally, you can have no more than $2,000 in savings for Medicaid to pay your long-term care costs. Partnership plans that offer to protect savings of up to $100,000, for example, will pay up to $100,000 in benefits and protect your assets. If you have savings of more than $100,000, you become responsible for your own long-term care costs until your savings are reduced to $100,000. At that point, Medicaid takes over the expenses.

Critics of long-term care insurance also note that most policies have a 90-day deductible, meaning most owners of long-term care insurance will receive no benefits until this time has passed. They argue that many who need long-term care use it for less than 90 days for rehabilitation in skilled nursing facilities, which Medicare covers. But who wants to play those odds? And the fact is, most people who need long-term care need it for at least a year or two. To be safe, I would recommend purchasing a zero day elimination policy. It might cost more, but it is worth it.

If you are considering long-term care insurance there are three options: a stand-alone long-term care policy, a fixed annuity with long-term care benefits, or a life insurance policy with a long-term care rider. Buying long-term care insurance is not a cookie cutter process. Your state insurance department can lead you to a licensed agent, and you can talk to him or her about what form best suits your needs. Because of the wide variations among the policies marketed by different companies, you should deal with an insurance agent who represents more than one carrier. **Do not**

rely upon any verbal promises by the agent. You must review any actual policy you are considering.

In the end, as with most insurance, deciding whether to buy at all is something of an educated guess. You may feel confident that you can handle the cost of long-term care on your own if you need it. I just ask that you not maintain a false sense of financial security. Why would you want to put millions of dollars at risk when you can afford the annual premium without changing your lifestyle? We take many gambles in our life, and I believe that long-term care insurance is a reasonable risk. Just start with a smaller policy that you can afford instead of a policy so cumbersome that it carries a risk that you may drop it. One of the swiftest ways to deplete an asset base is to get sick at the wrong time. Remember, this book is about keeping you out of a nursing home. Most people who live in such facilities have run out of money and are on Medicaid.

Reverse Mortgage

A reverse mortgage is a special type of home loan that lets you convert a portion of the equity that you built up over years of making mortgage payments on your home into cash. Unlike with a traditional home equity loan or second mortgage, you typically do not have to repay the loan until you no longer use the home as you principal residence or until you fail to meet the obligations of the mortgage. You do have to continue to pay for insurance and property taxes, however. If you fail to do that, the loan can be accelerated. (If you do have a problem paying your property taxes, most states have one or more property tax relief programs. For information on property tax relief in your state, contact the local agency to whom you pay your property taxes, your state department of revenue or taxation, or your nearest Area Agency on Aging.)

The technical name for a reverse mortgage is a Home Equity Conversion Mortgage (HECM). The HECM is the only reverse mortgage insured by the Federal Housing Administration (FHA), which is part of the U.S. Department of Housing and Urban Development (HUD). The FHA tells HECM lenders how much they can lend you based on your age and home value. The HECM program limits your loan costs, and the FHA guarantees that lenders will meet their obligations. Proprietary or privately insured reverse mortgages (those that are not FHA-insured HECM loans) virtually vanished from the marketplace during the recession. At present, only a small number of these products exist for very high-value homes. My discussion will therefore be limited to the HECM loan.

HECM loans are designed to provide additional housing finance options for homeowners aged 62 or older who own their homes outright, or who have low mortgage balances that can be paid off at closing with proceeds from the reverse loan. The dwelling must be a single family home, a two- to four-unit home with one unit occupied by the borrower, or a HUD-approved condominium or manufactured home that meets FHA requirements. The other stipulation is that you must live in the home. You may apply for an HECM even if you did not originally purchase your home with an FHA-insured mortgage. A reverse mortgage must be repaid in full under any of the following conditions: when the last surviving borrower dies or sells the home; if you allow the property to deteriorate (except for reasonable wear and tear), and you fail to correct the problem; if all borrowers permanently move to new principal residences; or if, because of physical or mental illness, the last surviving borrower fails to live in the home for 12 consecutive months.

This product has been a life saver for many of my clients. One client in particular, Bill, comes to mind. He was told that he had to either go home from the nursing home where he had rehabilitated with a full-time caregiver or go to an assisted living facility. Bill was *dead set on staying home with his Martin Crane chair and clicker. He had no money. His income was Social Security. But he had a house, paid in full, and his television set was there. This was important to him. There was no way for him to pay $6,000 a month unless he got a reverse mortgage.*

Bill's predicament was certainly not unique. Sometimes, it was the cost of medication that thrust a client into poverty and malnutrition, forcing her to choose between paying for life-saving drugs or food. Of course, one can use a reverse mortgage for happier scenarios (such as a cruise), and some of my clients have obtained reverse mortgages to pay for their long-term care insurance premiums. You can also use an HECM to purchase a primary residence if you are able to use cash on hand to pay the difference between the HECM proceeds and the sales price plus closing costs for the property you are purchasing. It is simply another tool that you can have in your arsenal if you own a home and qualify.

I have seen the depression lift from the shoulders of many clients when they realize that they can get money and not have to pay anything during their lifetime—no interest, no principal. The only objection is usually from an adult child who sees his inheritance disappear like a slippery salmon to the river from the hands of a hungry bear. Not to worry rapacious scion, when the home is sold or no longer used as a primary residence and the cash, interest, and other HECM finance charges are repaid, all remaining proceeds go to you. That is right! Any remaining equity can be transferred to heirs and, as an extra bonus, no debt is passed along to the estate or to the heirs.

The amount you may borrow will depend on a variety of factors such as: the age of the youngest borrower; the current interest rate; the lesser of the appraised value, the HECM FHA mortgage limit of $625,500, or the sales price; and whether you chose an HECM

Standard or HECM Saver as your initial mortgage insurance premium. As a general rule, if your home is valuable and you are very old, you can obtain a lower interest rate and a larger loan amount. Many online reverse mortgage calculators can provide you with an estimate of the amount of funds you can borrow.

You have a choice about how you receive the funds from the loan, and what you choose will depend on your own personal circumstances and needs. You can select from five different types of payment plans:

- **Tenure**, with equal monthly payments as long as at least one borrower lives in and continues to occupy the property as a principal residence.

- **Term**, with equal monthly payments for a fixed period of months selected.

- **Line of Credit**, with unscheduled payments or in installments, at times and in an amount of your choosing until the line of credit is exhausted.

- **Modified Tenure**, with a combination of line of credit and scheduled monthly payments for as long as you remain in the home.

- **Modified Term**, with a combination of line of credit plus monthly payments for a fixed period of months selected by the borrower.

But will the receipt of periodic payments or a lump sum disqualify you from Medicaid? It can. No matter how you take your money in a reverse mortgage, it is considered a loan. If you are looking at a financial statement, it is a liability, not an asset. The home is the asset. Many times we refer to the monthly payments incorrectly as monthly income, but neither the IRS nor Medicaid nor any other agency counts the funds from a reverse mortgage as taxable income or qualifying income. It is like taking a cash advance from a credit card. Just as you would then owe money to the credit card company, you owe money to the bank (with the key difference being that you do not have to pay it back immediately).

That said, the Medicaid or SSI guideline you need to be most cautious of is the cash on hand guideline, which stipulates you can have no more than $2,000 in your bank accounts. If you are taking $1,000 each month from a reverse mortgage and spending only $500, you will clearly exceed this amount within a few months. Once your balance exceeds $2,000, your assests will disqualify you from these programs. Likewise, if you choose to go the credit line route, you have to make sure that any lump sum you take out is used in the month you take it out so that it does not create a period of ineligibility.

You may also wonder why this product is so expensive. Limits on origination fees have not changed, but the willingness of lenders to reduce or even eliminate origination fees (and servicing fees) has changed dramatically. Since April 2010, some lenders have begun waiving or reducing origination fees on many of their loans. While some may offer these lower fees, you may pay in the end with a higher interest rate. And importantly, due to these high upfront costs, reverse mortgages are not an ideal option for anyone who may move or be transferred to a nursing home within a few years of taking one out, because the loan will come due if the homeowner does not live in the house for 12 consecutive months.

There are many reputable reverse mortgage lenders, but consumers should beware of phone and mail solicitations and always seek third party professional advice before signing any loan documents. In at least two states, Connecticut and Montana, housing finance agencies offer specialized reverse mortgage loans.

Deferred payment loans are also offered by some state and local government agencies. These allow consumers to repair or improve their homes by giving them one-time, lump sum advances for the specific types of repairs or improvements that each program allows. Typically these are limited to homeowners with low or moderate incomes. But again, for as long as you live in the home you are not required to pay these loans back.

Deferred payment loans go by many different names, so they may be difficult to find. Contact your city or county housing department or the nearest community action or community development agency. Also try your state housing finance agency or call your Area Agency on Aging (800-677-1116), or search online at www.eldercare.gov.

Another public sector version of the reverse mortgage is known as a property tax deferral (PTD) loan. Generally, these loans provide annual advances that can be used only to pay property taxes, and no repayment is required for as long as you live in the house. According to a 2007 AARP study, some type of PTD program is available in some or all of the following states: Arizona, California, Colorado, Florida, Georgia, Idaho, Illinois, Iowa, Maine, Maryland, Massachusetts, Michigan, Minnesota, New Hampshire, North Dakota, Oregon, Pennsylvania, South Dakota, Tennessee, Texas, Utah, Virginia, Washington, Wisconsin, Wyoming, and the District of Columbia.

Life Settlements

You might hear about opportunities to sell your life insurance policy for cash in a transaction known as a life settlement. A life settlement may also be called a senior settlement, and it involves selling an existing life insurance policy to a third party—a person or an entity other than the company that issued the policy—for more than the policy's cash surrender value but less than the net death benefit. Historically, if you owned a life insurance policy that you no longer wanted or needed, you generally had two choices: surrender the policy for its cash value or allow it to lapse.

You may recall a phenomenon with the AIDS movement in the 1980s whereby ordinary people and top-notch finance entrepreneurs purchased the insurance policies of those suffering from AIDS. This was a niche industry that involved viatical settlements of insurance policies. It was designed to provide a source of liquidity for AIDS patients and other terminally ill policyholders with life expectancies of less than two years These individuals, mostly men (92 percent) between the ages of 20 and 50 (88 percent), typically did not have children or spouses, and therefore did not have to worry about anyone else's welfare after their death. Because of their age, most were in the prime of their working lives, so they depended on earned income and did not have retirement money to draw on to pay their medical expenses.

Not unlike many seniors who face chronic illness, fixed incomes, and grown children who they do not have to "worry" about (although do we ever stop worrying about our children?), these victims faced terrible financial difficulties. Medical bills mounted up and their financial viability worsened as their ill health forced them to work less or not at all. There were so many willing to sell their policies that the fledgling viatical industry grew from only three investment companies in 1989 to at least fifty today. It is now a billion-dollar industry that includes life settlements. Like viatical settlements, whoever buys your policy as a life settlement acquires a financial interest in your death.

Those who purchase life settlements most often are institutions that hold the policies until maturity and collect the net death benefits, resell the policies, or sell interests in multiple, bundled policies to hedge funds or other investors. In return, the insured receives a lump sum payment. Sounds simple. However, the amount you will receive in the secondary market depends on a range of factors including your age and health, as well as the terms and conditions of your existing policy. The purchaser not only pays a lump sum for your policy, but also pays any additional premiums that might be required to support the cost of the policy for as long as you live. The Government Accountability Office found that insureds who completed life settlements received, on average, seven times more than the cash surrender value of their policies.[248]

If one of the factors driving your decision about a life settlement is a need for cash, you might want to see whether you can borrow against your policy. You might also be eligible for accelerated death benefits, which allow an individual with a long-term, catastrophic, or terminal illness to receive benefits on his or her policy prior to dying without incurring the potentially high costs associated with a life settlement.

When you sell a policy in the life settlement market, it stays in force and counts as part of your underwriting capacity—the maximum amount of exposure to loss an insurer can insure. Likewise, if you donate a policy to a charity or ownership is transferred to a family member, you no longer own the policy, yet it still counts as part of your underwriting capacity. Any of these scenarios could prohibit or limit you from purchasing additional insurance if you need it at a later date.

You should also know that a cash payment from a life settlement can have inadvertent financial consequences. For example, a lump sum payment can be taxable, depending on your circumstances. Moreover, as always, you really need to understand the impact that receiving a lump sum will have on your receipt of public benefits. If you currently receive Medicaid or SSI, a life settlement can negatively affect your eligibility. If you are considering this option, you should consult your attorney, accountant, or other legal or financial professional. These professionals will be able to help you reach a decision about whether a life settlement makes sense for you, and will also help you determine if you are getting a fair price and whether there are tax consequences associated with the transaction.

Today's life settlement market is highly sophisticated and regulated in more than 40 states affecting 90 percent of the U.S. population. Most states impose waiting periods of two to five years and require certain mandatory disclosures, the most important of which is agent and broker commissions. Commission disclosure is now a statutory requirement in New York and California—the two largest markets, accounting for nearly 40 percent of all settlements transacted in 2009—and is now an industry best practice required by all institutional funders.

Like with any other financial product, you must make sure that you are dealing with a reputable and licensed agent or company. Older adults are more susceptible to predatory practices and there are some very aggressive sales agents. I always recommend contacting your state insurance commissioner to ascertain the viability of a company and the product you are contemplating.

Patient Assistance Prescription Drug Programs

Patient Assistance Programs (PAPs) from drug manufacturers—also called indigent drug programs, charitable drug programs, or medication assistance programs—began back in the 1950s when the companies received government incentives. These programs help qualifying patients without prescription drug coverage get the medicines they need for free or nearly free. Most of the best known and most prescribed drugs can be found in these programs. There are over 250 PAPs (all of the major drug companies have them) and each has different guidelines. In general, you will qualify if you meet these three conditions:

1. You are a United States resident.
2. You are not insured for outpatient prescription drugs

(including Medicaid).

3. You have an income level that causes you to experience hardship when paying for retail prescriptions.

The exact definition of economic hardship varies with each PAP, though most adhere to a formula related to federal poverty guidelines. As a general rule, if your income is 200 percent of the federal poverty guideline or lower, then you will most likely qualify.

If you would like to find a program for yourself or a loved one, I suggest visiting each drug manufacturer's website. You can also check out a website that I stumbled upon called Needy Meds (www.needymeds.org). It is a non-profit information resource devoted to helping people find assistance programs to help them afford their medications and other costs related to health care. These programs can have long, complicated enrollment processes that may be overwhelming, but try not to be discouraged, because the financial payoff can be worth it.

If you are a Medicare beneficiary, your annual income is less than $16,245 for a single person or $21,855 for a couple, and you have limited assets, you may be eligible for extra help in paying for Medicare Prescription Drug Program premiums and other costs. This extra help can increase your cost savings by paying for part of the monthly premiums, annual deductibles, and prescription co-payments under the new prescription drug program. For questions, or to apply for extra help, call the Social Security Administration at 800-772-1213 or visit their website (www.socialsecurity.gov/i1020). You can also call your local Medicare/Medicaid Assistance Program at 800-803-7174.

Also, if you are a veteran and have completed 24 continuous months of active military service, you may be eligible for prescription drug coverage as part of your veteran benefits. Visit the Department of Veterans Affairs website (www.va.gov/healtheligibility/) or call 877-222-8387 for more information.

Aid and Attendance Benefits for Veterans

There are now over 25 million U.S. veterans eligible for VA benefits. Most believe they are only entitled to benefits if they were actually wounded or disabled while serving in the armed forces, but this is not true. More and more vets are realizing that VA special pensions exist, including the Aid and Attendance Pension. Even though local VA offices are not very forthcoming (or are totally ignorant) about it, it is not surprising that I am getting a lot of calls about this particular program.

Aid and Attendance is a "special monthly pension" available to wartime veterans or surviving spouses of wartime veterans. It provides a monthly stipend for in-home care, nursing home care, or care in an assisted living facility. As of January 2012, a single veteran qualifies for $1,704 a month, a married veteran qualifies for $2,020 a month, and a widowed surviving spouse can receive up to $1,094 a month. In order to receive the *maximum* aid, the veteran's countable income (including earnings, disability, retirement payments, interest and dividends, and net income from farming or a business) must be $0. Generally speaking, a veteran and his or her spouse may have up to $80,000 in assets to qualify for any Aid and Attendance benefit, though this is not a hard and fast rule. The eligibility worker will determine the assets the couple can have based on age and other factors. Public assistance, including SSI, is not included as countable income.

As a claimant, you must show that you require the "aid and attendance" of another person in order to perform some of the basic activities of daily living. The medical evidence must be provided by a physician. Additionally, if you reside in a facility, then the facility must also provide a letter stating that you reside there because you need assistance with the activities of daily living. The VA defines the need for aid and attendance as:

1. Requiring the aid of another person to perform at least
   two activities of daily living, such as grooming, transferring, eating, bathing, dressing or toileting;
2. Being blind or nearly blind; or
3. Being a patient in a nursing home.

Aid and Attendance is awarded on top of either the "service"
benefit or the "housebound" benefit. While there is <u>no</u> requirement
of a service-connected disability, the veteran or surviving spouse
must first be eligible for the "service" benefit, which requires the
veteran to have served at least 90 days of active military duty,
and at least one of those days had to be during wartime. The qualifying wars are: World War II (12/7/1941 through 12/31/1946);
the Korean Conflict (6/27/1950 through 1/31/1955); Vietnam
(8/5/1964 through 5/7/1975, or 2/28/1961 through 5/7/1975
for a veteran who served in the Republic of Vietnam during that
period); and the Gulf Wars (8/2/1990–current). The veteran has
to have received a discharge that was other than dishonorable.

There are many people who have served in capacities not
specifically in the Army, Navy, Air Force, or Marines who can get
these benefits. For example, I helped a family whose father was in
the Merchant Marines, and he was entitled to apply for and obtain
Aid and Attendance benefits.

There are financial eligibility requirements associated with any
VA pension, including for Aid and Attendance benefits. If you are
looking for a definitive answer on the amount of non-exempt
assets you can possess, you will be frustrated. If you look on the
Internet, you will see opinions that suggest that a single veteran
can have $80,000 and a widowed veteran is allowed $50,000 in
assets. In practice, however, the asset limits depend on your age
and the eligibility worker's mood. What you can count on is that
your home, a car, and personal effects are exempt and will not be
counted toward your asset limits. Unlike with Medicaid, there is

no recovery against your assets or estate after your death.

The VA will look at your gross income from all sources, less countable (unreimbursed) medical expenses. If your income after these adjustments is equal to or greater than the annual benefit amount, you (as the veteran or surviving spouse) are not eligible for benefits. Unreimbursed medical expenses include: long-term care or assisted living facility, health related insurance premiums (including for Medicare), diabetic supplies, private caregivers, incontinence supplies, prescriptions, and dialysis not covered by any other health plan. Only the portion of the unreimbursed medical expenses that exceeds 5 percent of the basic Maximum Annual Pension Rate (MAPR) may be deducted.

The following chart includes the set yearly income rate/annual pension Aid and Attendance and the maximum monthly benefit.

Aid and Attendance MAPR Category	Basic Pension MAPR	5% of Basic Pension MAPR	Annual Aid & Attendance Pension Rate
If you are...	Your basic pension MAPR is...	Subtract this amount from your medical expenses	To receive benefit, your countable yearly income must be less than...
A single veteran	$12,256 ($1,021 per mo.)	$613	$20,447 ($1,704 per mo.)
A veteran with spouse/ dependent	$16,051 ($1,337 per mo.)	$803	$24,239 ($2,020 per mo.)
Two veterans married to each other	$16,051 ($1,337 per mo.)	$803	$31,578 ($1,094 per mo.)
A surviving spouse	$8,219 ($684 per mo.)	$411	$13,138 ($1,094 per mo.)
A surviving spouse with one dependent	$10,759 ($896 per mo.)	$538	$15,673 ($1,306 per mo.)

Source: California Advocates for Nursing Home Reform
(http://www.canhr.org/factsheets/misc_fs/html/fs_aid_&_attendance.htm)

The California Advocates for Nursing Home Reform website offers the following example to explain the table:

Jim is a single veteran. He is disabled and needs help paying for care. His yearly income is $40,000 and he has $35,000 unreimbursed medical expenses this year.

- *His basic pension MAPR is $12,256; 5 percent of this amount (or $613) can be deducted from his eligible medical expenses.*
- *$35,000 medical expenses – $613 = $34,387 medical deduction*
- *Jim's $40,000 income – his $34,387 medical deduction = $5,613 countable income*

Jim's countable income is subtracted from the maximum annual Aid and Attendance Pension Rate to determine his benefit amount:

- *$20,447 (Aid and Attendance Rate)– $5,613 (countable income) = $14,834*

Jim's Aid and Attendance benefit would be $14,834 annually, or $1,236 monthly.

If you meet all the criteria for these benefits, you will still have to go through a painfully laborious and slow application process. It will typically take at least six months for approval. Just today I received a call in which a daughter told me that the VA has taken two years to process her father's application, citing bogus issues with his rating (an irrelevant red herring) and his marital status (another bogus issue). I feel confident that the VA really does not care if their ludicrous and intransigent position renders this man's 89-year-old wife destitute. The VA's own law states that applications for benefits for veterans and surviving spouses who are 70 or older are to be given priority, so if this describes you, you should state this in a cover letter accompanying the application and request the application process be expedited. Fortunately, the benefit is retroactive to the month after the application is submitted.

Please note that it is illegal for anyone to charge a fee for completing an application for Aid and Attendance benefits. While no one can charge a fee for actually preparing and submitting an application, an expert *can* charge a fee for assisting you to *qualify* for VA Aid and Attendance or Housebound benefits. Very few persons understand the "ins and outs" of the process, and it can be daunting. An expert can help you consider what care options are available to you, review the VA, Medicaid, and Medicare options and explain how each may apply to your circumstances, assess specific documents (including powers of attorney for property and health care matters, wills, and trusts), create a plan for the best use of your personal, financial, and family resources, and outline the consequences for income, capital gains, estate and/or gift taxes.

Keep in mind that some actions you might take to qualify for VA benefits can create a penalty period later when you need to qualify for Medicaid. Nevertheless, in the hands of an expert, and when properly integrated with other planning options, VA benefits might provide you with a tremendous financial boost. Only a state veterans affairs office, a Veterans Service Organization (VSO) such as VFW, or a licensed attorney certified by the Veterans Administration (like myself) can assist you with this. Veterans Service Organizations like the Veterans of Foreign Wars and the American Legion are private, non-profit groups that advocate on behalf of veterans. They play a critical role in advocacy and are often the initial contact in the community for veteran services. A VSO can help you fill out the application. To search for the nearest VSO visit the Veterans Affairs website (http://www.va.gov/ogc/apps/accreditation/index.asp) or consult Appendix C.

BEWARE. There are some companies that do not charge fees but are merely capitalizing on the volume of people seeking this benefit. They may suggest a product such as an annuity because they will make a huge commission off of it. These are insurance salesmen. It pays to get real professional advice from an elder law attorney or other noted resource before making any such purchase. When you are stuck in a product that does not serve you, you may feel like regurgitating your "free lunch."

To all of you who have served, I humbly thank you. It is only now that I am a mother that I recognize deeply what your service and sacrifice means to our country.

Medicaid

Medicaid (called "Medi-Cal" in California and "MassHealth" in Massachusetts) pays for medical care and long-term care in a *nursing home* for people with very low income and assets levels. While Congress and the federal Centers for Medicare and Medicaid Services (CMS) set out the main rules under which Medicaid operates, each state runs its own program. As a result, the rules are somewhat different in every state, although the framework is the same throughout the country.

In 2006, President Bush signed into law the Deficit Reduction Act of 2005 (DRA), and this cut nearly $40 billion over five years from Medicare, Medicaid, and other programs. Of greatest interest to the elderly and their families, the law placed severe new restrictions on the ability of the elderly to transfer assets before qualifying for Medicaid coverage of nursing home care. It made significant changes to the look-back period; the transfer penalty start date; the undue hardship exception; the treatment of annuities; community spouse income rules; home equity limits; the treatment of investments in continuing care retirement communities (CCRCs); promissory notes and life estates; and state long-term care partnership programs.

States have gradually adopted the new transfer rule. For the status of the rules in your state, and to understand whether you meet the prerequisites for the program, check with a qualified elder law attorney. California has yet to adopt the DRA. It is this fact that confines my advice about how the program works on a national level to generalities. But the most important item for me to cover is how giving away your assets could backfire and leave you homeless, because assets transferred during the look-back period will trigger a period of ineligibility.

The length of the ineligibility period is calculated by dividing the amount transferred by the average monthly cost of nursing home care in your area. In most states the look-back period is five years for transfers made after February 8, 2006 (except in California). If you are in need of care during that period and are now faced with no money, where will you go? Maybe your kids—to whom you made that transfer—will take you in? I have no idea why anyone would want to give away their money so that they can live in a nursing home, especially when doing so will result in a loss of dignity and a total depletion of one's resources. I *do* understand why people come to me when placement into a nursing home will result in spousal impoverishment, though there are some regulations in place that are designed to help avoid this.

A single person applying for Medicaid cannot have more than $2,000 in assets. A married couple cannot have more than $115,640, which includes $2,000 for the Medicaid applicant, and $113,640 for the applicant's spouse, in the form of the Community Spouse Resource Allowance (CSRA), which ensures that she does not become impoverished simply so the applicant can qualify for Medicaid. The spouse is also entitled to a Minimum Monthly Maintenance Needs Allowance (MMMNA) of $1,891.25 per month. The actual MMMNA can be higher depending upon the monthly shelter-related expenses incurred by the community spouse. The maximum income allowance during 2012 was $2,841. In the majority of states, if the community spouse's income does not equal as least $2,841 per month, she is allowed to keep all income that is solely in her name, plus half of all jointly owned income. Also, she may keep some of the nursing home spouse's income to get up to that minimum level. If the community spouse has high living expenses, she may appeal to keep more of the nursing home spouse's income—bringing her total minimum monthly income up to $2,841.

The institutionalized spouse must contribute all of his income toward the nursing home cost except for what is necessary for personal needs (typically less than $100 per month) and any amounts for health insurance, premiums, taxes and medical expenses not covered by Medicaid. This contribution of income toward his care is called his "liability."

Here is a list of assets that are considered exempt for eligibility purposes:

- The **applicant's principal residence**, as long as the equity is less than $786,000. In some states, the home will not be considered a countable asset for Medicaid eligibility purposes as long as the nursing home resident intends to return home; in other states, the nursing home resident must prove a likelihood of returning home. The home will also be excluded if the applicant's spouse resides in the home, or if a minor, blind, or disabled child resides in the home. This exclusion only applies if the property served as the recipient's primary residence prior to the nursing home admission.

- **One motor vehicle** is excluded, regardless of value, as long as it is used for transportation of the applicant or a household member. The value of an additional automobile may be excluded if it is needed for health or self-support reasons. (Check your state's rules.)

- **Prepaid funeral plans** and a small amount of **life insurance.**

- **Assets** that are considered "inaccessible" for one reason or another.

- **Personal possessions**, such as clothing, furniture, and jewelry.

If the home is sold during the Medicaid recipient's lifetime, the proceeds of the sale become an available asset. After the Medicaid recipient's death, if the home is included in the probate estate, then it will be a probate asset subject to creditor claims, including a claim by the state for reimbursement of Medicaid benefits. Some states have a right to place a lien on the Medicaid recipient's home to recover the value of benefits paid, which will be satisfied if the home is sold, whether during the recipient's lifetime or after death. Estate recovery is prohibited in certain instances when federal law deems that the needs of certain relatives for assets in the estate take precedence over Medicaid claims.[249] Specifically:

- During the lifetime of the surviving spouse, no matter where he or she lives;

- From a surviving child who is under age 21, or who is blind or permanently disabled (according to the SSI/Medicaid definition of "disability"), no matter where he or she lives;

- In the case of the former home of the recipient, when a sibling with an equity interest in the home has lived in the home for at least one year immediately before the deceased Medicaid recipient was institutionalized and has lawfully resided in the home continuously since the date of the recipient's admission; and

- In the case of the former home of the recipient, when an adult child has lived in the home for at least two years immediately before the deceased Medicaid recipient was institutionalized, has lived there continuously since that time, and can establish to the satisfaction of the state that he or she provided care that may have delayed the recipient's admission to the nursing home or other medical institution.

Again, because I do believe that a stay-at-home spouse can be impoverished by this system, it is very important to understand that there are legal mechanisms available to increase that individual's MMMNA allowance and CSRA. Before you embark upon applying for Medicaid, you must understand how your state defines assets and if any transfers of property are considered exempt (including those between spouses); you must also know the maximum amount of assets a person can retain and/or what court interventions are available to avoid spousal impoverishment. If you are in doubt as to whether you qualify for any of these benefits, contact your state Medicaid agency or a qualified elder law attorney. Alternatively, you can visit the Medicaid website (*www.medicaid.gov*).

Finally, if you want to make a go at staying in the community but you have limited means, there are some funds for home and community based-services. To qualify for either of the sources listed below, you must meet the Social Security Administration's definition of disability. Generally, that means proving that you are unable to work in any occupation and that the condition will last at least a year or is expected to result in death. If you meet these criteria you may be eligible for one or both of these:

- **Social Security Disability Income** is for workers younger than 65 who qualify for benefits.

- **Supplemental Security Income** guarantees a minimum monthly income for people who are age 65 or older, disabled, or blind, and who have very limited income and assets.

On February 11, 2010, the Social Security Administration (SSA) added early-onset (also called younger-onset) Alzheimer's to the list of conditions under its Compassionate Allowance Initiative, giving those with the disease expedited access to both Social Security Disability Insurance (SSDI) and Supplemental Security Income (SSI).

As you now know, there is a multitude of ways to finance your care. You are no longer operating in the dark and can breathe a sigh of relief. Depending on your financial situation, you may not have to choose any of the options I have described. Should the need arise, however, I hope that you find solace in the plethora of resoures available to you and your loved ones.

CHAPTER 12

We Used to Burn Our Bras Didn't We?

This final chapter speaks directly to those baby boomers who used to be politically active and who are now fat and content. It implores you to take a role in the political process that is so uniquely American and to force our leaders to pay attention to our needs as we age along the spectrum of time. There are big differences between boomers in terms of values, use of technology, work ethic, and respect and tolerance for others. What unifies you today is the need to understand how our government programs work and to understand our laws so that you can use them to your advantage. This is your right and duty. This chapter explains the laws that exist to protect all of us as we age. These laws can serve in concert with one another to keep us living independently but first, a little inspiration from our youth...

In the late 1960s, radical feminists used rhetoric and protest tactics to convey their disdain for the objectification of women.

They staged theatrical—and at times deliberately provocative—demonstrations (which they called "zap actions") to call attention to women's need for liberation. One such exhibition was the infamous protest against the 1968 Miss America beauty pageant. Protesters saw the pageant and its symbols as an oppression of women because of their emphasis on an arbitrary standard of beauty and the elevation of a choice of the "most beautiful girl in America" to a pedestal for public worship and commercial exploitation. Inspired by a statement by Germaine Greer that "bras are a ludicrous invention," 400 women from the New York Radical Women marched at the Atlantic City Convention Hall shortly after the Democratic National Convention. On September 7, 1968, a "Freedom Trash Can" was placed on the ground, and filled with bras, high-heeled shoes, false eyelashes, girdles, curlers, hairspray, makeup, corsets, magazines (such as Playboy), and other items thought to be "instruments of torture," accoutrements of enforced femininity.

Although a fire was never lit (a permit could not be obtained) and no burning occurred (contrary to the subsequent urban legend) this symbolic act called national attention to the emerging Women's Liberation Movement. The bra-burning tale was contrived by a female reporter who attempted to create an analogy to those who burned their draft cards in protest of the Vietnam War—a movement with established credibility. That telecast of the Miss America Pageant, with its media coverage of the protest, was one of the highest-rated programs of the year. Afterward, the women's movement gained momentum and the media increasingly took it seriously.

A few years earlier, the 1963 March on Washington for Jobs and Freedom, attended by some 250,000 people, was the largest demonstration ever seen in the nation's capital. The civil rights movement resulted in a host of legislative achievements, such as the passage of the Civil Rights Act of 1964, which banned discrimination based on "race, color, religion, or national origin" in employment practices and public accommodations. The Voting Rights Act of 1965 was also passed, followed shortly thereafter by the Immigration and Nationality Services Act of 1965. Additionally, in 1968, the Fair Housing Act banned discrimination in the sale or rental of housing. African Americans re-entered politics in the South, and across the country young people were inspired to action.

Simultaneous with the civil rights movement was the anti-war movement. In 1967, 300,000 protesters marched in New York City and 50,000 descended on the Pentagon, with more than 700 arrested in protest of the draft. Despite tactics organized by government agencies to inhibit the growth of the movement, as well as unsympathetic media coverage, by the end of 1967 public support for the war had dropped to barely one-third of the population. Further adding to the protestors' cause and the decline in support was the fact that, at its peak in 1968, 540,000 soldiers were at war, with more than 300 Americans being killed every week.

In October 1969, 3 million people participated in demonstrations as part of the Moratorium on the War. One month later, half a million protesters marched on Washington. The news media began to become more skeptical in its war coverage and mainstream churches and unions began to speak out more boldly. In 1970, after Nixon instituted the draft lottery and invaded Cambodia (when elected he promised to end the war), four Kent State University students were killed by National Guardsmen at an anti-war demonstration. Ultimately, a series of challenges to the draft ensued and, because it became so difficult for the Selective Service System to implement the convoluted regulations, the draft was ended. In January 1973, in response to a strong anti-war mandate, Nixon announced the effective end to U.S. involvement in Southeast Asia.

Why on earth would I dredge up these movements? They are in the past. What is their relevance here? It's simple: We are the individuals who these movements comprised. And we are the people who will suffer if we do not take charge of our futures now. We need to collectively understand what it will take to live in a safe and affordable environment when we are old, so that we can collectively act to make sure that it happens.

In the last forty years there have been fits and spurts of activism, yet today our country is more fractured than it has been in a long time. We have been through two wars that have left us with a new wave of young veterans suffering from psychological disturbances and lost limbs. We live in what many people refer to as the United States of Bank of America, which has created a huge schism between the wealthy and the poor. We bailed out the banking industry and the taxpayers are still suffering with the loss of their homes. Small businesses are suffering because of tightened lending practices. Since we, the taxpayers, bailed out the banks, they have seen record profits. In the third quarter of last year, Citigroup posted a net profit of $3.8 billion, a *74 percent increase* over the previous year when it received a taxpayer bailout.

Gas prices are higher than ever as oil companies make their biggest profits on record. And we just take it. Our children are being fed sludge by our public schools where teachers are facing pay cuts. These teachers already make 100 times less than hedge fund investors,[250] the top 25 of whom took in $22.07 billion in 2010. Thanks to a generous tax loophole, these billionaires paid a top tax rate of 15 percent instead of the maximum of 35 percent. Closing that loophole on just those 25 individuals would raise $4.4 billion, which is enough to rehire 126,000 laid-off teachers.

If this is something that bugs you...FIGHT! If any of this bugs you, fight. I am not a Tea Partier. In fact, my personal belief system is the polar opposite. However, I respect the fact that those in the Tea Party have passion and they assert it. I cannot find any movement in the twenty-first century that has had as much momentum and power. If you are sickened by the greed of the 1 percent, join the Occupy Wall Street movement or mentor those who could use the benefit of your wisdom.

If the prospect of living a sad existence at the end of your life bugs you, FIGHT.

As a first step, you need to be familiar with the laws that will protect you as you age, so let me explain them here.

Age Discrimination

As you grow older, you may face discrimination because someone believes you are no longer as capable as you once were. The Age Discrimination in Employment Act of 1967 (ADEA), enforced by the Equal Employment Opportunity Commission, is designed to protect individuals 40 years of age and older from discrimination on the basis of age in hiring, promotion, discharge, compensation, or terms, conditions, or privileges of employment. Section 188 of the Workforce Investment Act of 1998 (WIA) also prohibits discrimination against applicants, employees, and participants i*f*n WIA Title I financially assisted programs and activities, and programs that are part of the One-Stop system, on the grounds of age. WIA also prohibits discrimination on the grounds of race, color, religion, sex, national origin, disability, political affiliation, or belief, and for beneficiaries only, citizenship or participation in a WIA Title I financially assisted program or activity. Section 188 of WIA is enforced by the Civil Rights Center.

Hopefully, I have already convinced you in Chapter 11 that you deserve to transition from work to retirement on your own terms. Keep in mind that these laws are in place to ensure that you accomplish this. If you feel you have been discriminated against, you should consult a lawyer.

Disability Discrimination

Although a chronic physical or mental disability may occur at any age, the older we become, the more likely we are to develop disabling conditions. For example, less than 4 percent of children under 15 years old have severe disabilities, compared with 58 percent of people 80 years and older. The baby boom generation—those of us born between 1946 and 1964—will contribute significantly to the growth in the number of elderly individuals with disabilities who need long-term care and to the amount of resources required to pay for it.

I once represented a man who had been an airplane mechanic for a large international carrier. He was fired after 30 years of service. He had a perfect record and a history of awards and pay increases. He had Parkinson's disease. When he became disabled, he still wanted to work. They would not have it. In an email from the human resource department to my client's boss, it was the company's opinion that it could not continue to employ him because his disability made it impossible for my client to carry out his job functions. Just like that. No evidence, no physician evaluation, just pure ignorance. That was a good email. It made him a millionaire! I sued the company under The Americans with Disabilities Act (ADA), which guarantees equal opportunity for individuals with disabilities in employment, public accommodations, transportation, state and local government services, and telecommunications.

As I described in Chapter 7, if you have a disability, landlords may have to make certain *reasonable accommodations* or adjustments to the physical structure of your apartment so that you can have full use of your home. You can request a physical modification to accommodate your disability before moving into an apartment or during your tenancy. You should do this in writing. If you request a physical modification, you must show how the modification will help relieve the effects of your disability.

Right to Live in the Community

One June 22, 1999, the U.S. Supreme Court ruled in the case *Olmstead v. L.C. and E.W.* that the integration mandate of the Americans with Disabilities Act requires public agencies to provide services "in the most integrated setting appropriate to the needs of qualified individuals with disabilities." Disabled people who have been segregated in institutions have used this ruling to require states to provide services in the community. What is important to understand is that the Olmstead decision applies to *older adults* as well as their younger disabled counterparts. In other words, it applies to you.

Remember that the goal of this book is to *keep you out of a nursing home.* Therefore, you must understand that this law can and should be used to argue for more funding to support community-based programs for elders to move out of nursing homes and back into their communities, with services in place to sustain such moves. In some cases, a least restrictive environment can include the individual's own home. More funding is necessary to create tools to evaluate whether and when such a move is appropriate.

Historically, Medicaid long-term care expenditures have financed services delivered in nursing homes or other institutions. However, over the years, more and more resources have been allocated to home and community-based care. Community-based services are support services provided for people with disabilities and the elderly who live in their own homes and communities. Community-based services provide help for all aspects of a person's life and may include the following:

- Residential services and facilities, including supervised apartments or group homes;

- Personal assistance services, including assistive technology;

- Care planning, case management, and a comprehensive individualized plan, that includes a case manager, the person in need of services, and other people who support the individual;

- Day programs, including placement in activity centers and adult skills programs;

- Vocational services, including supported employment programs, job training and placement, and job coaching; and

- Other quality of life services, such as recreation, leisure, and transportation.

The principal means by which states provide these types of services is through another optional approach: home and community-based services (HCBS) waivers, which are set forth in section 1915(c) of the Social Security Act. States have to apply to the federal government for these waivers, which, if approved, give them greater flexibility in offering certain nonmedical and social services and supports that allow people to remain in the community. To receive waivers, states must demonstrate that the cost of the services to be provided is no more than what would have been spent on institutional care plus any other Medicaid services provided to an institutionalized individual.

States often operate several different waivers serving different population groups, and they often limit the size and scope of the waivers to help target their Medicaid resources and to control spending. The average costs for providing waivers and other home and community-based services are much lower than average costs for institutionalizing a person. However, the costs of these community-based services *do not* include other things that are necessary when a person lives in his or her home or in a community-based setting, such as costs for housing, meals, and transportation, as well as the additional costs and burden for family and other informal caregivers. The proportion of Medicaid long-term care spending devoted to home and community-based services varies widely. Some states have taken advantage of Medicaid HCBS waivers to develop extensive home and community-based services, while others have traditionally relied more heavily on institutional and nursing facility services.

Medicaid is an important component of states' abilities to meet the Olmstead mandate. While Medicaid spending for home and community-based services is growing, these are largely optional benefits that states may or may not choose to offer, and as a result, they vary widely in the degree to which they cover them as part of their Medicaid programs. Consequently, the ability of Medicaid-eligible people with disabilities to access care in home and community-based settings also varies widely from state to state and even from community to community. But the scope of the ADA and the Olmstead decision is *not* limited to Medicaid beneficiaries or to services financed by the Medicaid program. The ADA and the Olmstead decision apply to all qualified individuals with disabilities, regardless of age. This is a very important point that should not be forgotten, particularly now when states' Medicaid budgets are in such peril.

The sad reality is that few states are seriously evaluating older nursing home residents to determine their degree of readiness to move from nursing homes to the least restricted environments, and this constitutes a failure on the part of state agencies to implement the Olmstead Act. Additionally, in most states, the demand for HCBS waiver services has exceeded what is available and has resulted in long waiting lists.

If, in your newly rekindled zest for advocacy, you choose to take this issue on, you need to know more about the specific components of the Olmstead Act and how they impact frail elders:

- If an individual's application for community-based service is denied, the individual has the right to re-apply (Social Security Act 1902 (a) (3)). Agencies must have due process procedures in place for clients who are denied services. Sometimes denying services involves refusing to take the client's name because of the long waiting list; other times it might involve telling the client that the agency is not accepting applications or referrals at this time.

- Older disabled persons are covered under Freedom of Choice. Freedom of Choice means that a Medicaid client can choose between receiving services in the community or in an institutional setting. If an elder meets the institutional care requirement, he has the right to select where he will receive that care. Furthermore, states cannot impose limits on the number of Medicaid eligible clients they serve. States have faced and continue to face lawsuits for imposing limits in the number of beds available to Medicaid eligible individuals (Social Security 1902(a)(3)).

- Federal courts have ruled that Social Security Act 1902 (a)(8) bars states from wait listing individuals for entitled Medicaid services if they have been approved. Services should be delivered in a timely fashion. A waiting list or a priority assessed client list that is not moving and is keeping elders for months with no in-home services is not considered delivering services in a timely fashion.

- All type of services should exist in all geographical locations. Social Security 1902 (a)(10) states that Medicaid

services need to be available on a comparable basis to all
eligible individuals. Offering a waiver in one part of the
state and not in another is a violation of this rule. This
involves Medicaid waiver programs like Consumer
Directed Care, PACE, Nursing Home Diversion and
assisted living facilities. Waivers should be available in
all geographical areas of the state if the state possesses
such a waiver program.

- Advocates should evaluate if a particular state has
  placed more restrictive financial eligibility criteria on
  frail elders than on individuals with disabilities. If this is
  the case, this is also a violation of the Social Security
  Act regulations, which mandate the same eligibility
  criteria for everyone.

Affordable Care Act

If the Affordable Care Act is not eviscerated by a changing of
the guard in the 2012 election, nearly half of the 8.6 million uninsured Americans between the ages of 50 and 64 will gain access
to medical care through subsidized coverage. Low-income older
adults will maintain access to preventative health care and screenings. The phasing out of the donut hole has already saved 5
million elders and disabled individuals $3.2 billion. The preserva-
tion on the ban to deny health coverage to those with pre-existing
conditions means that they will enter the Medicare system in
healthier condition, thus saving money in the long term. The
Affordable Care Act provides more opportunities to age in place
with community support.

Even if the Act remains intact, there are still potential problems
for younger uninsured elders. Originally, the law required states
to expand access to their Medicaid programs to more uninsured

individuals or lose all of the federal support they receive for their program. The court upheld this expansion, but it also limited the federal government's ability to sanction the states that did not comply. Some state governors have already said that they will not expand Medicaid, leaving a lot of money that could be spent on millions of their poorest citizens without health coverage. We must pressure state officials to take up the federal government's offer to fund the Medicaid expansion.

Family Caregiving

FMLA, also known as the Family Medical Leave Act, is a piece of federal legislation that was passed in 1993. It allows you 12 weeks, either consecutive or intermittent, of unpaid work leave to address medical concerns involving yourself or specified loved ones. Upon completion of the leave you are eligible to return to your same employment position or one that is equivalent. It provides you with job protection for the duration of your leave based on certain qualifications. You can use FMLA to care for an immediate family member—including parents or a spouse—with a serious health condition. Importantly, you cannot use FMLA leave to care for a father-in-law or mother-in-law.

Generally, you are eligible for FMLA if you have been employed for at least one year and 1,250 hours within the last 12 months by a business with 50 or more employees within a 75-mile radius or a public agency, including a school or a state, local or federal employer. You may also be entitled to paid leave under your employer's short-term disability program. You may be able (or your employer may require you) to use your sick time or vacation time while you are on FMLA leave.

Five states—California, Hawaii, New Jersey, New York, and Rhode Island—as well as Puerto Rico have Temporary Disability Insurance programs to provide some pay if you are out of work due to your own serious health condition. California and New Jersey provide a more comprehensive paid family leave program allowing for payment if you need time off to care for a family member or to bond with your new child. Washington State recently passed a paid parental leave program that will go into effect pending funding.

For more information you can check out the Department of Labor website (www.dol.gov).

The Older Americans Act

Congress passed the Older Americans Act (OAA) in 1965 in response to concern on the part of policymakers about a lack of community social services for older persons. The original legislation established authority for grants to states for community planning and social services, research and development projects, and personnel training in the field of aging. The OAA created the National Aging Network comprising the Administration on Aging on the federal level, State Units on Aging, and Area Agencies on Aging at the local level.

The need for these programs serving older adults and caregivers cannot be overstated. Senior hunger and unemployment among people age 55 and older continue to rise. There are 10,000 baby boomers turning 65 each day, so needs will only continue to grow. Individuals over the age of 85, the fastest growing segment of the aging population, are the most vulnerable older adults who most need the long-term services, support, and protection from abuse, neglect, and financial exploitation that are provided under Older Americans Act programs.

In the face of the growing needs of seniors and the disabled, grant allotments for senior jobs programs have been cut, as have funds for vulnerable rights protections through the Long-Term

Care Ombudsman program. Federal funding levels for nutrition and supportive services are also in jeopardy, as they have not kept pace with inflation or the growth of our aging population. And, according to the National Council on Aging, since 2004 the Older Americans Act appropriations have lagged behind the rising costs of fuel, commodities, and wages. There are waiting lists for home-delivered meals and other vital services.

Elder Justice

The Elder Justice Act—included in the 2010 health care reform law—is designed to coordinate federal and state efforts to test ways to prevent elder abuse, neglect, and exploitation. Just when everyone thought that the Act would go down with the ship, on June 14, 2012, Health and Human Services (HHS) Secretary Kathleen Sebelius announced a $5.5 million funding opportunity for states and tribes to test ways to prevent elder abuse, neglect, and exploitation. Funding for this program is essential to all of us who desire to stay independent and live with dignity. If you are robbed by an unscrupulous moron, you will be stuck having to live in a nursing home (and the government will be stuck with the tab).

Nursing Home Reform

I know that you were paying very careful attention to every detail of this book and that you hung on every word plunked down from my brain to this page. Just in case some of my brilliance was lost, however, in my criticism of the nursing home industry were clues about what you can do to push proprietors into acting more responsibly. Many of the specific problems that need our attention tie to the conditions that nursing home residents are confronted with on a daily basis, whether they are aware of the problems or not. For example:

- Older frail adults should not be housed with the mentally ill population. We need to support funding for housing this distinct group of individuals.

- Criminal background checks for facility workers should not be optional and should not be left to the discretion of the states. Make your state lawmakers aware of the dangers of these practices.

- Get behind campaigns (or start one) that attempt to force the nursing home industry to stop overmedicating "problem" residents.

- Demand higher mandatory staffing ratios. Demand laws that prevent dubious hospital transfers of frail residents. These individuals are more likely to have feeding tubes inserted, spend time in intensive care in their last months of life, have severe bedsores, or be enrolled in hospice late (three days or less before death).

Other specific problems that desperately need our attention stem from the very limited avenues of recourse that nursing home residents have when they encounter problems. With this in mind, I encourage you to:

- Speak out against damage caps involved in suing facilities for wrongdoing. Residents and their families should have the right to appropriate compensation when they have been victimized by neglect.

- Also speak against arbitration agreements, which hog tie residents who have been harmed by the facilities that purport to care for them.

- Make a case for clear lines of nursing facility ownership; finding the responsible party should not be like looking for Waldo.

- Be a harbinger of cultural change in nursing homes by demanding that the interpretation of regulations and the way that government surveyors cite noncompliant homes be consistent and coherent.

- Advocate for continuity in how states determine specific deficiency citations so that there is a reliable, uniform method for individuals to check out the history of any facility.

- Investigate whether your state has passed laws that provide explicit criminal penalties for various forms of elder abuse. If your state has not passed these laws, become a voice in favor of them.

Miscellaneous Causes

Your activism need not—and should not—be limited to nursing homes. If we, as a generation, are to age with dignity and grace, there are numerous other causes that deserve our energy and focus as well. Here are some other ways that I implore you to get involved:

- Advocate for abolishment of mandatory retirement in all industries; it is ageist.

- Understand that if employers are allowed to continue exporting jobs overseas rather than jumping through hoops to attract older American workers, you may not have a choice about when you retire or return to the workforce once you do retire. Understand that legislative changes must be made to allow older workers to continue to work, or to return to work, without financial penalty (e.g., changes in Social Security, pension plans, IRS regulations).

- Support mass transportation measures in your community so that older adults won't be isolated if they lose their licenses. (It is good for the environment too!)

- Get involved in Alzheimer's research. The National Institutes of Health (NIH) spends $3 billion a year on research about AIDS, which affects around 1 million people in the United States. Nearly 5.5 million Americans are believed to have Alzheimer's, yet the disease receives just under $500 million a year for research. The government funds more nutrition research than it does Alzheimer's research. You can find out how to get more involved by going to the Alzheimer's Association website (www.alz.org).Fight for enhanced funding for Older Americans Act services, and advocate for improvements to the law through the next reauthorization. To learn how to get more involved, visit the Administration on Aging website (www.aoa.gov) and type "OAA" into the search box.

- Get involved in efforts to ensure that financial elder abuse is not a recurrent theme. Make sure that family members or financial planners do not rip off the elderly—or if they do, that they get raked over the coals.

- Buy long-term care insurance.

- Exercise and eat right.

BE PREPARED!
And thank you for listening.
Love,
Susan

ABOUT THE AUTHOR

Susan was born on the south side of Chicago and moved to Morton Grove after the Martin Luther King riots in 1968. She received her Bachelor's degree in Speech Pathology and Audiology from Illinois State University and after moving to California, her Law Degree from Loyola Law School of Los Angeles. She was a civil rights attorney for most of her career advocating for elderly and disabled clients.

She received her Master's degree in Gerontology from the University of Southern California after teaching as an Elder Law Professor at Loyola Law School and serving as in-house counsel for a major nursing home corporation based in Southern California.

As one of only a few elder law attorneys in the United States with a Master's Degree in gerontology, Susan is often referred to as the "guru" of the aging industry. Her popular elder care seminar tour, "Raising UP Your Parents" has been attended by thousands of adult children and seniors in search of answers to elder care challenges. She is a highly sought after lecturer for associations and corporations throughout the U.S.

Susan continues to practice as a geriatric care manager and elder law attorney in California, and consults with families throughout the U.S. over the phone.

List of Resources

Hopefully this book has given you some great ideas about how to take control of your future, so that your golden years are spent in the environment that *you* choose. Throughout the text, I've intentionally given you many resources and directed you to numerous websites and organizations. To make it easier for you to find them, I have also listed them here—along with a few additional ideas—so that you can find what you need easily.

Books and websites can be incredible resources as you plan your own or your loved one's next steps in this journey, but sometimes you want to talk with a real, live person. I have worked one-on-one with clients for many years, both in person and by telephone. If you would like to hire me to work with you on a more personal basis, please contact me through my website (www.susanbgeffen.com). I can help you navigate a full range of elder care issues, or focus in on specific concerns.

I also encourage you to visit the educational resource section of my website for an even more detailed list of where you can turn for guidance and information as you travel the road ahead.

NAVIGATING THE PROCESS

I offer many useful tools and resources that I have developed through my work as an elder care consultant and elder law attorney. I have listed them in this section, together with the names and contact information of larger organizations that can connect you with other professionals doing similar work.

www.susanbgeffen.com

At my website you will find access to many helpful tools, including:

> The resources section of my site (www.susanbgeffen.com/resources), where you can read and download lots of great information, presented in even more detail than what's contained in this book.

> My e-newsletter (www.susanbgeffen.com/newsletter), which includes articles I have written about current events affecting baby boomers and seniors.

> Information about my seminars, "Raising UP Your Parents" (www.susanbgeffen.com/seminars).

> My contact information should you wish to communicate directly with me.

My YouTube Channel

www.youtube.com/susanbgeffen

On my YouTube channel you will find many entertaining and educational videos where I speak about important issues and conduct interviews with clients and experts in the aging industry.

Susan's Picks *(Coming Soon!)*
www.susanbgeffen.com/susanspicks
Finding companies you can trust can be challenging, especially when so much is at stake. Susan's Picks lists companies that have been screened by my staff and I. Simply insert your zip code and the service or product you want. If your zip code is not yet listed, check back for updates.

Raising UP Your Parents
www.susanbgeffen.com/seminars
I designed this seminar for adult children of aging parents and seniors. It is the most comprehensive of its kind, covering many of the elder care topics I address in this book along with some that I do not. These seminars will be offered nationally soon; check my website for updates.

National Association of Professional Geriatric Care Managers
www.caremanager.org
If you are interested in hiring an elder care consultant, this nonprofit website can direct you to a professional in your area.

National Association of Area Agencies on Aging (N4A)
202-872-0888
www.n4a.org
N4A is an umbrella organization for local Area Agencies on Aging. The website has a search tool that will allow you to locate nearby agencies that can help you connect with a wide range of services and information useful to you and your family.

Veterans Service Officers
http://www.va.gov/ogc/apps/accreditation/index.asp
Veterans Service Officers (VSOs) are professional veterans affairs advocates and are often the initial contact in the community for veteran services. Follow the link above to search for a VSO in your area.

CHOOSING A PLACE TO LIVE
I've given you a lot of advice about how to choose the best long-term care option for yourself. When it comes time to make a choice, you'll want the most up-to-date, current, and carefully selected information possible. The links in this section are designed to give you just that.

Nursing Home Compare
www.medicare.gov/nhcompare
This site provides detailed information about every Medicare- and Medicaid-certified nursing home in the country.

Joint Commission on the Accreditation of Healthcare Organizations (JCAHO)
www.jointcommission.org
Use the JCAHO "Quality Check" to find facilities that have been accredited by the Joint Commission, indicating higher staffing levels and higher quality of care.

Continuing Care Accreditation Commission (CCAC)
202-783-7286
www.carf.org/Programs/AS/
CCAC is part of the National Institutes of Health's National Institute on Aging. The organization accredits a full range of long-term care solutions, including continuing care retirement communities (CCRCs), nursing homes, adult day services, assisted living, home and community services, and dementia and stroke programs.

Agency for Healthcare Research and Quality (AHRQ)
www.ahrq.gov
The AHRQ is run by the U.S Department of Health and Human Services. Its website will provide details about your state's approach to regulation, survey practices, and special initiatives.

Assisted Living Federation of America (ALFA)
www.alfa.org
ALFA monitors assisted living statues in every state, and provides current regulations on its website. The site also provides research articles and public policy documents that are relevant to older adults.

National Center for Assisted Living (NCAL)
www.ahcancal.org
Part of the American Health Care Association, the National Center for Assisted Living monitors trends and statistics related to long-term care.

U.S. Department of Housing and Urban Development (HUD)
www.hud.gov
HUD's site includes many links with details about various senior housing options, as well as information about reverse mortgages. Visit the link above and type "seniors" into the search box.

RESOURCES FOR AGING AT HOME

If you have made the decision to stay in your own home, at some point you are likely to need to make some adjustments so that you are comfortable and safe. The resources in this section will help you do that.

Americans With Disabilities Act (ADA)

www.ada.gov

The ADA website describes the rights of individuals with disabilities in employment, public accommodations, transportation, state and local government services, and telecommunications.

National Adult Day Services Association (NADSA)

www.nadsa.org

This website will provide you with checklists and guidance that will help you find the right Adult Day Center for yourself or a loved one.

Program of All Inclusive Care for the Elderly (PACE)

www.cms.hhs.gov/pace/pacesite.asp

PACE programs provide comprehensive long-term services for Medicaid and Medicare recipients, usually at home. The website provides a directory of PACE organizations nationwide.

U.S. Department of Labor

www.dol.gov

Among other things, the Department of Labor website provides details about what is covered under the Family & Medical Leave Act (http://www.dol.gov/dol/topic/benefits-leave/fmla.htm), which can be especially important if you need to care for a loved one at home.

National Transit Hotline

800-527-8279

The National Transit Hotline maintains a list of federally funded providers of transportation services for the elderly and disabled.

Red Cross

1-800-RED-CROSS

www.redcross.org

Contact the Red Cross to request a copy of its 32-page guide titled *Disaster Preparedness for Seniors by Seniors*, which will help you prepare for emergencies.

Beacon Hill Village

www.beaconhillvillage.org

Beacon Hill Village is an innovative neighborhood-based organization that enables and empowers older adults to maintain full, healthy lives while continuing to live at home. Its publication, *The Village Concept: A Founder's Manual*, provides information about how to start similar organizations.

INSURANCE AND OTHER FINANCIAL MATTERS

The financial aspects of growing older can be complicated and overwhelming. I hope I have taken some of the stress out of the equation with all of the information I presented in the book. That being said, I understand that a book is often not an adequate substitute for a professional who can assist you directly. I continue to work with fee-based clients who hire me to guide them when things get too complicated or stressful.

I am available for telephone consultations on all of the issues that I have covered here. *In California*, I am licensed to provide legal services such as estate planning, Medi-Cal Asset Protection planning, and assistance with acquiring Veterans Aid and Attendance benefits. Visit my website (www.susanbgeffen.com) for a complete list of the services I offer.

Medicare
www.medicare.gov
The Medicare website provides information about costs and coverage. Of particular interest is the section on prescription drug coverage.

Medicaid
www.medicaid.gov
The Medicaid website can help you determine whether your state has a waiver program that will pay for assisted living care, adult family home care, in-home care, and/or nursing home placement.

Centers for Medicare and Medicaid Services (CMS)
www.cms.gov
CMS can help you coordinate your Medicare and Medicaid benefits.

Social Security Administration
800-772-1213
www.socialsecurity.gov/i1020
If you are enrolled in a Medicare prescription drug plan, you may be able to get assistance with paying for your medication. Visit this link to see if you are eligible.

U.S. Department of Veterans Affairs
www.va.gov

The website of the Department of Veterans Affairs will provide you with comprehensive information about your rights and entitlements as a veteran of the United States Armed Forces. For example, you can apply for health benefits (http://www.va.gov/healthbenefits/
or 877-222-8387)
and home loans (http://www.benefits.va.gov/ homeloans/
or 800-827-1000).

U.S. Department of Housing and Urban Development (HUD)
www.hud.gov
HUD's site includes information about reverse mortgages.

Needy Meds
www.needymeds.org
This non-profit information resource will direct you to programs that can help you afford your medications and other costs related to health care.

MENTAL AND PHYSICAL HEALTH
Maintaining your mental and physical health is as important as maintaining your financial security. The resources listed in this section will help you do just that.

National Institute on Aging (NIA)
www.nia.nih.gov
The National Institute on Aging provides many publications (most of them free) that address a wide range of topics related to aging and mental health, including depression
(http://www.nia.nih.gov/ health/publication/depression)
and sexuality in later life.
(http://www.nia.nih.gov/health/publication/ sexuality-later-life).

National Institutes of Health (NIH)
www.nih.gov
The website of the NIH can direct you to many resources related to healthy aging (http://health.nih.gov/category/SeniorsHealth), including the relationship between sleep and healthy aging (http://health.nih.gov/topic/SleepDisorders).

AARP (formerly the American Association of Retired Persons)
www.aarp.org
AARP's website offers wonderful resources and advice about all aspects of growing older, including a comprehensive section on issues related to sex and intimacy (http://www.aarp.org/home-family/sex-intimacy/).

American Association of Sexuality Educators, Counselors, and Therapists (AASECT)

www.aasect.org

The website of this professional association can connect you with a licensed therapist or counselor who specializes in issues related to sexuality. The site also offers an extensive list of other resources addressing the topic.

National Adult Protective Services Association (NAPSA)

www.apsnetwork.org

NAPSA was founded to improve the quality and availability of protective services for adults who are abused, neglected, or exploited and are unable to protect their own interests. If you know a vulnerable person who may be in an abusive situation, you can report it to NAPSA and have it investigated.

National Suicide Prevention Lifeline

1-800-273-TALK (8255)

This suicide prevention telephone hotline is funded by the U.S. government and provides free, 24-hour assistance.

National Hopeline Network

1-800-SUICIDE (784-2433)

Call this toll-free telephone number to receive suicide crisis support at any hour of the day.

Appendix A

Nursing Home Checklist

Checklists can help you evaluate the nursing homes that you call or visit. Use a new checklist for each home you call or visit. Then, compare the scores. This will help you select a nursing home that is a good choice for you or your relative.

Nursing Home Name: _____

Date Visited: _____

Address: _____

1. Basic Information

1. Is the facility Medicare certified?   ____(yes)   _____(no)

2. Is the facility Medicaid certified?   ____(yes)   _____(no)

3. Is this a skilled nursing facility?   ____(yes)   _____(no)

4. Is the facility accepting new patients?   ____(yes)   _____(no)

5. Is there a waiting period for admission?   ____(yes)   _____(no)

6. Is a skilled bed available to you?   ____(yes)   _____(no)

Useful Tips

- Generally, skilled nursing care is available only for a short period of time after a hospitalization. Custodial care is for a much longer period of time. If a facility offers both types of care, learn if residents may transfer between levels of care within the nursing home without having to move from their old room or from the nursing home.
- Nursing homes that only take Medicaid residents might offer longer term but less intensive levels of care. Nursing homes that don't accept Medicaid payments may make a resident move when Medicare or the resident's own money runs out.
- An occupancy rate is the total number of residents currently living in a nursing home divided by the home's total number of beds. Occupancy rates vary by area, depending on the overall number of available nursing home beds.

2. Nursing Home Information

Is the home and the current administrator licensed?: ____(yes) ____(no)
Does the home conduct background checks on all staff?:____(yes) ____(no)
Does the home have special services units?: ____(yes) ____(no)
Does the home have abuse prevention training?: ____(yes) ____(no)

Useful Tips

- **LICENSURE**: The nursing home and its administrator should be licensed by the state to operate.
- **BACKGROUND CHECKS:** Do the nursing home's procedures to screen potential employees for a history of abuse meet your state's requirements? Your state's ombudsman program might be able to help you with this information.
- **SPECIAL SERVICES:** Some nursing homes have special service units like rehabilitation, Alzheimer's, and hospice. Learn if there are separate waiting periods or facility guidelines for when residents would be moved on or off the special unit.
- **STAFF TRAINING:** Do the nursing home's training programs educate employees about how to recognize resident abuse and neglect, how to deal with aggressive or difficult residents, and how to deal with the stress of caring for so many needs? Are there clear procedures to identify events or trends that might lead to abuse and neglect, and on how to investigate, report, and resolve your complaints?
- **LOSS PREVENTION:** Are there policies or procedures to safeguard resident possessions?

For Sections 3 through 6, give the nursing home a grade from one to five.
One is worst, five is best.

3. Quality of Life

	Worst				Best
1. Residents can make choices about their daily routine. Examples are when to go to bed or get up, when to bathe, or when to eat.	1	2	3	4	5
2. The interaction between staff and patient is warm and respectful.	1	2	3	4	5
3. The home is easy to visit for friends and family.	1	2	3	4	5
4. The nursing home meets your cultural, religious, or language needs.	1	2	3	4	5
5. The nursing home smells and looks clean and has good lighting.	1	2	3	4	5

6. The home maintains comfortable temperatures.	1	2	3	4	5
7. The resident rooms have personal articles and furniture.	1	2	3	4	5
8. The public and resident rooms have comfortable furniture.	1	2	3	4	5
9. The nursing home and its dining room are generally quiet.	1	2	3	4	5
10. Residents may choose from a variety of activities that they like.	1	2	3	4	5
11. The nursing home has outside volunteer groups.	1	2	3	4	5
12. The nursing home has outdoor areas for resident use and helps residents to get outside.	1	2	3	4	5

3. TOTAL: _____
(Best Possible Score: 60)

4. Quality of Care

	Worst				Best
1. The facility corrected any quality of care deficiencies that were in the state inspection report.	1	2	3	4	5
2. Residents may continue to see their personal physician.	1	2	3	4	5
3. Residents are clean, appropriately dressed, and well groomed.	1	2	3	4	5
4. Nursing home staff respond quickly to requests for help.	1	2	3	4	5
5. The administrator and staff seem comfortable with each other and with the residents.	1	2	3	4	5
6. Residents have the same care givers on a daily basis.	1	2	3	4	5
7. There are enough staff at night and on weekends or holidays to care for each resident.	1	2	3	4	5

8. The home has an arrangement for emergency situations with a nearby hospital.　　1　2　3　4　5

9. The family and residents councils are independent from the nursing home's management.　　1　2　3　4　5

10. Care plan meetings are held at times that are easy for residents and their family members to attend.　　1　2　3　4　5

4. TOTAL: _____
(Best Possible Score: 50)

Useful Tips

• Good care plans are essential to good care. They should be put together by a team of providers and family and updated as often as necessary.

5. Nutrition and Hydration (Diet and Fluids)

	Worst				Best

1. The home corrected any deficiencies in these areas that were on the recent state inspection report.　　1　2　3　4　5

2. There are enough staff to assist each resident who requires help with eating.　　1　2　3　4　5

3. The food smells and looks good and is served at proper temperatures.　　1　2　3　4　5

4. Residents are offered choices of food at mealtimes.　　1　2　3　4　5

5. Residents' weight is routinely monitored.　　1　2　3　4　5

6. There are water pitchers and glasses on tables in the rooms.　　1　2　3　4　5

7. Staff help residents drink if they are not able to do so on their own.　　1　2　3　4　5

8. Nutritious snacks are available during the day and evening.　　1　2　3　4　5

9. The environment in the dining room encourages residents to relax, socialize, and enjoy their food.　　1　2　3　4　5

5. TOTAL: _____
(Best Possible Score: 45)

Useful Tips

- Ask the professional staff how the medicine a resident takes can affect what they eat and how often they may want something to drink.
- Visit at mealtime. Are residents rushed through meals or do they have time to finish eating and to use the meal as an opportunity to socialize with each other?
- Sometimes the food a home serves is fine, but a resident still won't eat. Nursing home residents may like some control over their diet. Can they select their meals from a menu or select their mealtime?
- If residents need help eating, do care plans specify what type of assistance they will receive?

6. Safety

	Worst				Best
1. There are handrails in the hallways and grab bars in the bathrooms.	1	2	3	4	5
2. Exits are clearly marked.	1	2	3	4	5
3. Spills and other accidents are cleaned up quickly.	1	2	3	4	5
4. Hallways are free of clutter and have good lighting.	1	2	3	4	5
5. There are enough staff to help move residents quickly in an emergency.	1	2	3	4	5
6. The nursing home has smoke detectors and sprinklers.	1	2	3	4	5

6. TOTAL: _____
(Best Possible Score: 30)

Useful Tips Relating to Information in Nursing Home Compare

Nursing Home Compare contains summary information about nursing homes from their last state inspection. It also contains information that was reported by the nursing homes prior to the last State inspection including nursing home and resident characteristics. If you have questions or concerns about the information on a nursing home, you should discuss them during your visit. This section contains useful tips and questions that you may want to ask the nursing home staff, family members and residents of the nursing home during your visit.

Nursing Home Compare Information on Results of Nursing Home Inspections

- Bring a copy of the Nursing Home Compare inspection results for the nursing home. Ask whether the deficiencies have been corrected.
- Ask to see a copy of the most recent nursing home inspection report.

Nursing Home Compare Information on Resident and Nursing Home Characteristics

1. For the Measure: Residents with Physical Restraints
- Does it appear that there is sufficient staff to assist residents who need help in moving or getting in and out of chairs and bed?
- Ask the Director of Nursing who is involved in the decisions about physical restraints.
- When physical restraints are used, do the staff remove the physical restraints on a regular basis to help residents with moving, and with activities of daily living?
- Do the staff help residents with physical restraints to get in and out of bed and chairs when they want to get up?
- Do staff help residents with physical restraints to move as much as they would like to?

2. For the Measure: Residents with Pressure (Bed) Sores
- Ask the staff how they identify if a resident is at risk for skin breakdown. Ask them what they do to prevent pressure sores for these residents.
- Ask the staff about the percentage of their residents that have pressure sores and why.
- Do you see staff helping residents change their positions in wheelchairs, chairs, and beds?

3. For the Measure: Residents with Bowel and Baldder Incontinence
- Does the nursing home smell clean?
- Ask the staff what steps they take to prevent bowel and bladder incontinence for residents who are at risk.

4. For the Measure: Residents Who Are Very Dependent in Eating
- Look at your response to Question 2 in Section 5 above.
- Observe residents who need help in eating. Are they able to finish their meals or is the food returned to the kitchen uneaten?

5. For the Measure: Residents Who Are Bedfast
- Ask the Director of Nursing how staff are assigned to care for these residents.

6. For the Measure: Residents with Restricted Joint Motion
- Ask the Director of Nursing how the nursing home cares for residents with restricted joint motion.
- Do the residents get help with getting out of chairs and beds when they want to get up?

7. For the Measure: Residents with Unplanned Weight Gain or Loss
- Look at your responses to Questions 2, 3, 4, 5, 8, and 9 in Section 5 above.

8. For the Measure: Residents with Behavioral Symptoms
- What management and/or medical approaches for behavioral symptoms are being used by the nursing home?
- How does staff handle residents that have behavioral symptoms such as calling out or yelling?
- Ask whether residents with behavioral symptoms are checked by a doctor or behavioral specialist.
- Ask whether staff get special training to help them to provide care to residents with behavioral symptoms.

Nursing Home Compare Information on Nursing Staff

Caring, competent nursing staff who respect each resident and family member are very important in ensuring that residents get needed care and enjoy the best possible quality of life. Adequate nursing staff is needed to assess resident needs, plan and give them care, and help them with eating, bathing and other activities. Some residents (e.g., those who are more dependent in eating or who are bedfast) need more help than other residents depending on their conditions.

The combinations of registered nurses (RNs), licensed practical and vocational nurses (LPNs/LVNs), and certified nursing assistants (CNAs) that nursing homes may have vary depending on the type of care that residents need and the number of residents in the nursing home.

- Look at your responses to Questions 2 and 5 in Section 3 above and Questions 4, 5, and 10 in Section 4 above. Also look at your responses to Questions 2 and 7 in Section 5 above.
- Are nursing staff members courteous and friendly to residents and to other staff?
- Do nursing staff respond timely to resident's calls for assistance such as help getting in and out of bed, dressing and going to the bathroom?
- Observe meal times. Do all residents who need assistance with eating get help? Do staff give each resident enough time to chew food thoroughly and complete the meal?
- Which nursing staff members are involved in planning the resident's individual care? (Are they the same ones who give the care to residents?)
- Ask questions about staff turnover. Is there frequent turnover among certified nursing assistants (CNAs)? What about nurses and supervisors, including the Director of Nursing and the Administrator? If staff changes frequently, ask why.
- While the number of nursing staff is important to good care, also consider other factors, such as education and training. How many registered nurses (RNs) are on the staff, and how many available on each shift? What kind of training do certified nursing assistants (CNAs) receive? How does the nursing home ensure that all staff receives continuing education and keeps their knowledge and skills up-to-date?

Source: Medicare.gov

Appendix B

Home Care Licensing Guidelines by State

ALASKA
License Required?: NO
Certification Required?: Yes – by state
Who To Contact: Department of Health & Social Services
Telephone: 907-269-3666
Details: Certification based on experience, knowledge of Administrator

ALABAMA
License Required?: NO
Certification Required?: NO

ARKANSAS
License Required?: NO
Certification Required?: NO

ARIZONA
License Required?: NO
Certification Required?: NO

CALIFORNIA
License Required?: NO
Certification Required?: NO

COLORADO
License Required?: YES
Who To Contact: Licensure Customer Assistance Line
Telephone: 303-692-2836

CONNECTICUT
License Required?: YES
Certification Required?: NO
Who To Contact: Dept. of Consumer Protection
Telephone: 860-713-6100

DISTRICT OF COLUMBIA
License Required?: YES
Certification Required?: NO
Who To Contact: District of Columbia: Health Regulation & Licensing
Administration

Telephone: 202-724-8800
Details: called Home Care Agency

DELAWARE
License Required?: YES
Certification Required?: NO
Who To Contact: Office of Health Facilities Licensing & Certifications
Telephone: 302-995-8521
Additional: Personal Assistance Services Agencies must be licensed to provide services in Delaware
Details: All questions and request for application should be made by contacting the office by phone.

FLORIDA
License Required?: YES
Certification Required?: NO
Who To Contact: Lenore Lawry, Home Care Unit
Telephone: 840-414-6010
Details: Click on Homemaker Companion Services Application for registration and application information

GEORGIA
License Required?: YES
Certification Required?: NO
Who To Contact: Office of Regulatory Services, Dept of Human Resources
Telephone: 404-657-1509

HAWAII
License Required?: NO
Certification Required?: NO

IOWA
License Required?: NO
Certification Required?: NO

IDAHO
License Required?: NO
Certification Required?: NO

ILLINOIS
License Required?: YES
Certification Required?: NO
Who To Contact: Department of Healthcare and Family Services
Telephone: 217-782-1200
Details: Info on Private Duty Website is current

INDIANA
License Required?: YES
Certification Required?: NO
Who To Contact: Connie Wright
Telephone: 317-233-7742
Details: called Personal Care Agencies; is licensed and regulated

KANSAS
License Required?: NO
Certification Required?: NO

KENTUCKY
License Required?: NO
Certification Required?: NO

LOUISIANA
License Required?: YES
Certification Required?: NO
Who To Contact: Department of Health and Hospitals Division of Health Standards
Telephone: 225-342-0138
Details: call the division for a licensing packet

MASSACHUSETTS
License Required?: YES
Certification Required?: YES
Who To Contact: Office of Labor and Workforce Development, 617-626-6970

MARYLAND
License Required?: YES
Certification Required?: NO
Who To Contact: Department of Heath and Mental Hygiene, Office of Health Care Quality
Telephone: 410-402-8040
Details: Residential Service Agency license

MAINE
License Required?: YES
Certification Required?: NO
Who To Contact: Licensing and Certification for Personal Care Ageny
Telephone: 800-262-2232
Additional:
Details: Info on Private Duty Website is current

MICHIGAN
License Required?: NO
Certification Required?: NO

MINNESOTA
License Required?: YES
Certification Required?: NO
Who To Contact: Department of Health
Details: Info on Private Duty Website is current

MISSOURI
License Required?: NO
Certification Required?: NO

MISSISSIPPI
License Required?: NO
Certification Required?: NO

MONTANA
License Required?: NO
Certification Required?: NO

NORTH CAROLINA
License Required?: YES
Certification Required?: NO
Who To Contact: Division of Health Service Regulation
Telephone: 919-855-4620
Details: called Home Care Licensing; listed under Acute and Home Care Licensure & Certification Services

NORTH DAKOTA
License Required?: YES
Certification Required?: NO
Who To Contact: Department of Human Services
Telephone: 800-472-2622
Details: Qualified Service Provider (Agency Provider) Handbook with links to forms and explanation of standards to meet.

NEBRASKA
License Required?: YES
Certification Required?: NO
Who To Contact: Department of Health & Human Services, Div of Public Health Licensure Unit
Telephone: 401-471-4923
Details: Call department for licensing application

NEW HAMPSHIRE
License Required?: YES
Certification Required?: NO
Who To Contact: Bureau of Health Facilities Administration
Telephone: 800-852-3345 ext 4592
Details: Info on Private Duty Website is current

NEW JERSEY
License Required?: YES
Certification Required?: NO
Who To Contact: Department of Law & Public Safety Division Consumer Affairs
Telephone: 973-504-6370
Details: Info on Private Duty Website is correct; new online information

NEW MEXICO
License Required?: NO
Certification Required?: NO

NEVADA
License Required?: YES
Certification Required?: NO
Who To Contact: Bureau of Healthcare Quality & Compliance - Rosemary Helsing
Telephone: 775-687-4475
Details: License type is PCA; checklist of requirements available onsite.

NEW YORK
License Required?: YES
Certification Required?: NO
Who To Contact: Department of Health Div of Home & Community Based Care
Telephone: 518 -408-1629
Details: Licensed Home Care Services Agency (LHCSA) Online Permit Assistance and Licensing

OHIO
License Required?: NO
Certification Required?: NO

OKLAHOMA
License Required?: YES
Certification Required?: NO
Who To Contact: Department of Health Protective Health Services
Telephone: 405-271-6576
Details: Application is pdf on website; call office for more information

OREGON
License Required?: YES
Certification Required?: NO
Who To Contact: Department of Health Services Public Health Division
Telephone: 971-673-1222

PENNSYLVANIA
License Required?: YES
Certification Required?: YES/Register
Who To Contact: Department of Health Division of Home Health
Telephone: 877-724-3258
Details: Info on Private Duty Website is current

RHODE ISLAND
License Required?: YES
Certification Required?: NO
Who To Contact: Department of Health Office of Facilities Regulation
Telephone: 401-222-2566
Details: Info on Private Dute Website current except for name of RN

SOUTH CAROLINA
License Required?: YES
Certification Required?: YES

SOUTH DAKOTA
License Required?: NO
Certification Required?: NO

TENNESSEE
License Required?: YES
Certification Required?: NO
Who To Contact: Department of Mental Health & Developmental Disabilities
Telephone: 615-532-6590

TEXAS
License Required?: YES
Certification Required?: NO
Who To Contact: Department of Aging & Disability Services
Telephone: 512-438-3011
Details: HCSSAs must be licensed; complete pre-survey computer-based training

UTAH
License Required?: YES
Certification Required?: NO

Who To Contact: Department of Health Facility Licensing
Telephone: 800-662-4157
Details: At website select Rules, select R432-700 (Home Health Agency Rule) select Sec. 30 Home Health-Personal Care Service Agency

VIRGINIA
License Required?: YES
Certification Required?: NO
Who To Contact: Department of Health Office of Licensure & Certification, Acute Care Division
Telephone: 804-367-2102

VERMONT
License Required?: NO
Certification Required?: NO

WASHINGTON
License Required?: YES
Certification Required?: NO
Who To Contact: Department of Health Facilities Services Licensing
Telephone: 360-236-2905

WISCONSIN
License Required?: NO
Certification Required?: NO

WEST VIRGINIA
License Required?: NO
Certification Required?: NO

WYOMING
License Required?: NO
Certification Required?: NO

Appendix C

Congressionally Chartered Veterans Service Organizations (By Date of Charter)

Navy Mutual Aid Association (Jul. 28, 1879)

The American Red Cross (Jan. 5, 1905)

The American Legion (Sept. 16, 1919)

National Amputation Foundation, Inc. (1919)

American War Mothers (Feb. 24, 1925)

Disabled American Veterans (June 17, 1932)

Veterans of Foreign Wars (May 28, 1936)

Marine Corps League (July 4, 1937)

United Spanish War Veterans (April 22, 1940)

Navy Club of the United States of America (June 6, 1940)

American Veterans Committee (1944)

American Defenders of Bataan and Corregidor (Mar. 21, 1946)

AMVETS (American Veterans) (July 23, 1947)

American G.I. Forum (March 1948)

Military Chaplains Association of the USA (Sept. 20, 1950)

Legion of Valor of the USA, Inc. (July 4, 1955)

Congressional Medal of Honor Society (July 14, 1958)

Veterans of World War I (July 18, 1958)

Military Order of the Purple Heart (Aug. 26, 1958)

Blinded Veterans Association (Aug. 27, 1958)

Blue Star Mothers of America, Inc. (June 1960)

National Association for Black Veterans, Inc. (July 1969)

Paralyzed Veterans of America (Aug. 11, 1971)

Swords to Plowshares: Veterans Rights Organization (Dec. 23, 1974)

Veterans of the Vietnam War, Inc. (May 5, 1980)

Gold Star Wives of America, Inc. (Dec. 4, 1980)

Italian American War Veterans (Nov. 20, 1981)

U.S. Submarine Veterans, Inc. (Nov. 20, 1981)

National Veterans Legal Services Program, Inc. (1981)

American Ex-Prisoners of War (Aug. 10, 1982)

Women's Army Corps Veterans Association (Oct. 30, 1984)

American Gold Star Mothers, Inc. (June 12, 1984)

Polish Legion of America (June 23, 1984)

Catholic War Veterans (Aug. 17, 1984)

Jewish War Veterans (Aug. 21, 1984)
Pearl Harbor Survivors (Oct. 7, 1985)
Vietnam Veterans of America (May 23, 1986)
Army and Navy Union (Nov. 6, 1986)
Non-Commissioned Officers Association of America (April 6, 1988)
National Association of County Veterans Service Officers, Inc. (June 1990)
Military Order of the World Wars (Oct. 23, 1992)
The Retired Enlisted Association (Oct. 23, 1992)
Fleet Reserve Association (Oct. 23, 1996)
Air Force Sergeants Association (Nov. 18, 1997)
National Association of State Directors of Veterans Affairs (NASDVA) (N/A)
Women Airforce Service Pilots of World War II (N/A)

Other Veterans Service Organizations and Military Associations
Air Force Association
Association of the United States Army
Association for Service Disabled Veterans
Berlin Airlift Veterans Association
Enlisted Association of National Guard
National Association of County Veteran Service Officers
National Association of Uniformed Services
National 4th Infantry (IVY) Division
National Guard Association of the United States
Reserve Officers Association
The Retired Military Officers Association

Other Veterans' Links of Interest
2011 Edition of the Federal Benefits for Veterans, Dependents and Survivors
Veterans News and Information Services
Troops To Teachers
Gov Benefits

Memorial Links
World War II Veterans Memorial
Korean War Veterans Memorial
Vietnam War Veterans Memorial
The Women's Memorial

Source Notes

[1] Catherine Hawes, "Elder Abuse in Residential Long-Term Care Settings: What Is Known and What Information Is Needed?," in *Elder Mistreatment: Abuse, Neglect and Exploitation in Aging America—Supporting Papers*, eds. Richard J. Bonnie & Robert B. Wallace (Washington, DC: National Academy Press, 2003), 446–447.

Minority Staff Special Investigations Division, *Abuse of Residents Is a Major Problem In U.S. Nursing Homes* (Washington, DC: US House of Representatives, 2001).

[2] Charlene Harrington, Helen Carrillo, Brandee Woleslagle Blank, and Teena O'Brian, *Nursing Facilities, Staffing, Residents and Facility Deficiencies, 2004 through 2009* (San Francisco: UCSF, 2010).

[3] Charlene Harrington, Brian Olney, Helen Carrillo, and Taewoon Kang, "Nurse Staffing and Deficiencies in the Largest For-Profit Nursing Home Chains and Chains Owned by Private Equity Companies," *Health Services Research* 47, no. 1 (2012). doi: 10.1111/j.1475-6773.2011.01311.x

[4] The technical name for this profession is geriatric care management, but many are not familiar with that term so I prefer elder care consultant. You can find geriatric care managers in your city by going to the National Association of Professional Geriatric Care Managers website (http://www.caremanager.org/).

[5] Metlife Mature Market Institute, "Long-Term Care IQ Survey Shows Limited Knowledge About Long-Term Care" (Press Release) (New York: Metlife, 2009).

[6] Jeffrey Pfeffer and Robert Sutton, *The Knowing-Doing Gap: How Smart Companies Turn Knowledge into Action* (Boston: Harvard Business School Press, 2000).

[7] Alvin Toffler, "The Future as a Way of Life," *Horizon Magazine* 7, no. 3 (Summer 1965).

[8] Charles R. Pierret, "The 'Sandwich Generation': Women Caring for Parents and Children," *Monthly Labor Review* 129, no. 9 (2006): 3.

[9] Watson Wyatt Worldwide, "From Baby Boom to Elder Boom, Providing Health Care for an Aging Population (Washington, DC: Watson Wyatt, 1996).

[10] Richard Schulz and Scott R. Beach, "Caregiving as a Risk Factor for Mortality: The Caregiver Health Effects Study, *JAMA* 282, no. 23 (1999): 2259–60.

[11] American Health Assistance Foundation, "The Facts on Alzheimer's Disease." Available at http://www.ahaf.org/alzheimers/about/understanding/facts.html.

[12] According to a UC San Francisco study of nursing home residents, 80 percent died within one year of admission. The average age of study participants at admission was just over 83 years, and the average length of stay prior to death was just

under 14 months. The median stay, however, was just five months, and 53 percent of the nursing home residents in the study pool died within six months. Men, married people, and wealthy people died faster than their female, unmarried, and poorer counterparts. (See: Anne Kelly, Jessamyn Conell-Price, Kenneth Covinsky, Irena Stijacic Cenzer, Anna Chang, W. John Boscardin, and Alexander K. Smith, "Length of Stay for Older Adults Residing in Nursing Homes at the End of Life," *Journal of the American Geriatrics Society* 58, no. 9 (2010): 1701–1706.)

[13] ElderWeb, "Urbanization Created More Problems For The Elderly." Available at http://www.elderweb.com/book/1900-1929/urbanization-created-more-problems-elderly.

[14] James Finneran, "Families Around the World," *United Nations Chronicle* 31, no. 1 (1994): 46–47.

[15] In recent years, younger adults have begun moving away from rural areas. At the same time, many baby boomers have begun a rural retirement migration to escape the fast pace of the city and for recreational opportunities. At least one third of these boomers move to join adult offspring or other relatives and live out their lives in these communities. However, when these "migrants" get older and need more complex health services, they very often go back to urban areas. In communities where there is the political will and capacity to adjust to an "old" age structure, where an obstetrics ward—closed because the younger population has diminished—can be converted to an acute care unit, aging in the boonies may be a great alternative to the expensive city life.

[16] Martin Schultz, "Divorce Patterns in Nineteenth-Century New England," *Journal of Family History* 15, no. 1 (1990): 101–115.

[17] Medicine Encyclopedia, "Nursing Homes: History." Available at http://medicine.jrank.org/pages/1243/Nursing-Homes-History.html#ixzz19vn5ypfq.

[18] Kevin C. Flemming, Jonathan M. Evans, and Darryl S. Chutka, "Symposium on Geriatrics: A Cultural and Economic History of Old Age in America," *Mayo Clinic Proceedings* 78 (2003): 914–921.

[19] Carole Haber and Brian Gratton, *Old Age and the Search for Security* (Bloomington, IN: Indiana University Press, 1994).

[20] Jennifer Gimler Brady, "Long Term Care Under Fire: A Case For Rational Enforcement," *Journal of Contemporary Health Law Policy* 18, no. 1 (2001): 6–7.

[21] Medicine Encyclopedia, "Nursing Homes: History." Available at http://medicine.jrank.org/pages/1243/Nursing-Homes-History.html#ixzz19vn5ypfq.

[22] Robert N. Butler, *Why Survive? Being Old in America.* (New York: Harper and Row, 1975).

[23] Institute of Medicine, *Improving the Quality of Care in Nursing Homes* (Washington, DC: Institute of Medicine, 1986), as quoted in *Beverly Health & Rehabilitation Services v. Thompson*, 223 F. Supp. 2d 73, 78 (D.D.C. 2002).

[24] Ibid.

[25] Omnibus Reconciliation Act of 1987, Pub. L. No. 100–203, 101 Stat. 1330.

[26] Ibid (citing *42 USC. § 1395i-3*(g), 1396r(g) (2000)).

[27] Ibid., p. 108.

[28] Administration on Aging, *The National Elder Abuse Incidence Study: Final Report* (Washington, DC: Administration on Aging, 1998). Available at http://www.aoa.gov/eldfam/Elder_Rights/Elder_Abuse/AbuseReport_Full.pdf. See also Ellen F. Netting, Ruth N. Ellen Paton, and Ruth Huber, "The Long-Term Care Ombudsman Program: What the Complaint Reporting System Can Tell Us," *Gerontologist* 32 (1992): 843–849.

[29] Betty S. Black, Peter V. Rabins, and Pearl S. German, "Predictors of Nursing Home Placement Among Elderly Public Housing Residents," *Gerontologist* 39, no. 5 (1999): 559–568.

[30] Catherine A. Fullerton, Thomas G. McGuire, Zhanlian Feng, Vincent Mor, and David C. Grabowski, "Trends in Mental Health Admissions to Nursing Homes: 1999–2005," *Psychiatric Services* 60, no. 7 (2009): 965–71.

[31] John Gever, "Nursing Homes 'Dumping Grounds' for Mentally Ill," *MedPage Today*, March 23, 2009. Available at http://www.medpagetoday.com/Psychiatry/GeneralPsychiatry/13380.

[32] Samuel E. Simon, Debra J. Lipson, and Christal M. Stone, "Mental Disorders Among Non-Elderly Nursing Home Residents," *Journal of Aging & Social Policy* 23, no 1 (2011): 58–72.

[33] Janet Rehnquist, Inspector General, Department of Health and Human Services, *Nursing Home Deficiency Trends and Survey and Certification Process Consistency (03 OEI-02-01-00600)* (Washington, DC: Department of Health and Human Services, 2003). Available at http://oig.hhs.gov/oei/reports/oei-02-01-00600.pdf.

[34] Nicholas G. Castle, John Engberg, and Aiju Men, "Variation in the Use of Nursing Home Deficiency Citations," *Journal for Healthcare Quality* 29, no. 6 (2007): 12–23.

[35] Mark S. Lachs, Christianna S. Williams, and Shelley O'Brien, "The Mortality of Elder Mistreatment," *JAMA* 280, no. 5 (1998): 428–32.

[36] National Center on Elder Abuse, *The National Elder Abuse Incidence Study: Final Report* (Washington, DC: US Department of Health and Human Services, 1998). Available at http://www.aoa.gov/AoARoot/AoA_Programs/Elder_Rights/Elder_Abuse/docs/ABuseReport_Full.pdf.

[37] Calvin H. Hirsch, Sara Strattan, and Roberta Loewy, "The Primary Care of Elder Mistreatment," *Western Journal of Medicine* 170, no. 6 (1999): 353–358.

[38] Sidney M. Stahl, "The Need for a National Investment in Research on Elder Abuse and Neglect" (Short Paper), *Elder Justice: Medical Forensic Issues Relating To Abuse And Neglect (Roundtable)* (Washington, DC: US Department of Justice, 2001).

[39] See Laura A. Dummit, *Aggregate Medicare Payments Are Adequate Despite Bankruptcies*, GAO/T-HEHS-00-192 (Washington, DC: GAO, 2000) and Debra Sparks, "Nursing Homes: On the Sick List," *Business Week*, July 5, 1999.

[40] Ibid.

[41] Michael L. Rustad, "Neglecting The Neglected: The Impact of Noneconomic Damage Caps On Meritorious Nursing Home Lawsuits," *The Elder Law Journal* 14, no. 2 (2006): 345.

[42] Ibid., 343–344.

[43] Ibid.

[44] Ibid., 356.

[45] Minority Staff Special Investigations Division, *Nursing Home Conditions In Los Angeles County: Many Homes Fail to Meet Federal Standards for Adequate Care* (Washington, DC: US House of Representatives, 2003): 2 (as cited in Michael L. Rustad, "Neglecting the Neglected," *The Elder Law Journal* 14, no. 2 (2006): 357).

[46] Florida Policy Exchange Center on Aging, *Informational Report of the Task Force on Availability and Affordability of Long-Term Care for the Florida Legislature in Response to House Bill 1993* (Tampa, FL: University of South Florida, 2001).

[47] Greg Groeller and Bob LaMendola, Skyrocketing Suits Spur Crisis in Care Residences Plagued with Financial Dilemmas, *South Florida Sun-Sentinel*, March 4, 2001.

[48] Ibid.

[49] Ibid., 382.

[50] Catherine Pearsall, "Forensic Biomarkers Of Elder Abuse: What Clinicians Need To Know," *Journal of Forensic Nursing* 1, no. 4 (2005): 182–186.

[51] California Advocates for Nursing Home Reform, *Much Ado About Nothing: Debunking the Myth of Frequent and Frivolous Elder Abuse Lawsuits Against California's Nursing Homes*, (San Francisco: CANHR, 2003). Available at http://www.canhr.org/reports/2003/CANHR_Litigation_Report.pdf.

[52] Ibid.

[53] Americans for Insurance Reform, *Medical Malpractice Insurance: Stable Losses/Unstable Rates* (New York: Americans for Insurance Reform, 2002).

[54] Charlene Harrington, Helen Carrillo, Brandee Woleslagle Blank, and Teena O'Brian, *Nursing Facilities, Staffing, Residents and Facility Deficiencies, 2004 Through 2009* (San Francisco: UCSF, 2010).

[55] Andrew Schneider, "Neglected to Death: Preventable Deaths in Nursing Homes," *St. Louis Post-Dispatch*, October 14, 2002.

[56] 31 U.S.C. Section 3729 (1988).

[57] Larry D. Lahman, "Bad Mules: A Primer on the Federal False Claims Act," *Oklahoma Bar Journal* 76, no. 12 (2005): 901. Available at http://www.okbar.org/obj/articles_05/040905lahman.htm.

[58] David Hoffman, "The Role of the Federal Government in Ensuring Quality of Care in Long-Term Care Facilities," *Annals of Health Law* 6 (1997): 147–56.

[59] David Hoffman, "The Federal False Claims Act as a Remedy to Poor Care," *False Claims Act and Qui Tam Quarterly Review* 6 (1996): 17–22. Available at http://www.taf.org/PDF/jul96qr.pdf.

[60] Jack A. Meyer and Stephanie E. Anthony, *Reducing Health Care Fraud: An Assessment of the Impact of the False Claims Act* (Washington, DC: Taxpayers Against Fraud, 2001). Available at http://www.taf.org/publications/PDF/925_taf.pdf.

[61] Steven Pelovitz, Statement to the Senate Special Committee on Aging, *Nursing Home Bankruptcies*, Hearing, September 5, 2000. Available at http://aging.senate.gov/events/hr57sp.pdf.

[62] See Catherine Hawes, "Elder Abuse in Residential Long-Term Care Settings: What Is Known and What Information Is Needed?," in *Elder Mistreatment: Abuse, Neglect and Exploitation in Aging America—Supporting Papers*, eds. Richard J. Bonnie & Robert B. Wallace (Washington, DC: National Academy Press, 2003), 446–447; Minority Staff Special Investigations Division, *Abuse of Residents Is a Major Problem In U.S. Nursing Homes* (Washington, DC: US House of Representatives, 2001).

[63] Ruth Kilduff, "The Liability Crises: Reasons, Realities and Remedies," *Seniors Housing Research Notes*, May 15, 2001.

[64] Dee McAree, "Carving Out a Lucrative Niche," *National Law Journal*, July 26, 2004, S15.

[65] Richard S. Biondi, "Nursing Home Liability Insurance," *The Actuarial Digest* 20, no. 4 (2001).

[66] On average, for-profit nursing homes have 32 percent fewer nurses and 47 percent higher deficiencies than non-profit nursing homes. See Charlene Harrington et al., "Does Investor Ownership of Nursing Homes Compromise the Quality of Care?," *American Journal of Public Health* 91, no. 9 (2001): 1452–1455.

[67] Richard S. Biondi, "Nursing Home Liability Insurance," *The Actuarial Digest* 20, no. 4 (2001).

[68] Karl Pillemer and David Moore, "Highlights from a Study of Abuse of Patients in Nursing Homes," *Elder Abuse and Neglect* 2, no. 1 (1990): 5–30.

[69] Andrea Peterson, "Nursing Homes Face Nursing Crunch: Wave of Consumer Lawsuits Pushes Costs of Malpractice Insurance Higher; Some Doctors Stop Seeing Seniors," *Wall Street Journal*, June 3, 2004.

[70] David Stevenson, Statement to the Senate Special Committee on Aging, *Liability in Long Term Care*, Hearing, July 15, 2004. Available at

http://aging.senate.gov/events/hr127ds.pdf. Stevenson's empirical study of nursing home litigation claims suggests "that attorneys mobilized in this area in the mid-1990s and the claims and the size of recoveries have grown substantially in recent years" (p. 2).

[71] David G. Stevenson and David M. Studdert, "The Rise of Nursing Home Litigation: Findings From a National Survey of Attorneys," *Health Affairs* 22, no 2 (2003): 219, 221–22.

[72] Brian Burwell, David Stevenson, Eileen Tell, and Michael Schaefer, *Recent Trends in the Nursing Home Liability Insurance Market* (Washington, DC: US Department of Health and Human Services, 2006). Available at http://aspe.hhs.gov/daltcp/reports/2006/NHliab.pdf.

[73] Terry Carter, "Tort Reform Texas Style: New Laws and Med-Mal Damage Caps Devastate Plaintiff and Defense Firms Alike," *ABA Journal*, October 2006.

[74] Florida Health Care Association, *Report of the Joint Select Committee on Nursing Homes*, March 1, 2004. Available at http://www.fhca.org/members/legis/legis2004/2004jscnh.pdf.

[75] Charles Duhigg, "At Many Homes, More Profit and Less Nursing," *New York Times*, September 23, 2007.

[76] Richard J. Bonnie and Robert B. Wallace, "Introduction," in *Elder Mistreatment: Abuse, Neglect and Exploitation in Aging America—Supporting Papers*, eds. Richard J. Bonnie & Robert B. Wallace (Washington, DC: National Academy Press, 2003).

[77] See Marie-Therese Connolly, "Federal Law Enforcement In Long Term Care," *Journal of Health Care Law and Policy*, 4, no. 2 (2002): 230. The United States might pursue prosecutions implicating quality or failure of long-term care under a variety of federal criminal statutes. For example:

    Failure to perform a public duty:
        18 U.S.C. Sec 4 (2001), misprision of a felony
    Fraud or false statements:
        18 U.S.C. Sec 1347 (2001), which includes health care fraud incorporating the definition from 18 U.S.C. Sec 1346
        18 U.S.C. Sec 1035 (2001), false statements about health care matters
        18 U.S.C. Sec 1001 (2001), false statements
    Conspiracy:
        18 U.S.C. Sec 371 (2001)
    Obstruction:
        18 U.S.C. Sec 1516 (2001), obstruction of a federal audit
        18 U.S.C. Sec 1505 (2001), obstruction of proceedings before a grand jury
        18 U.S.C. Sec 1510 (2001), obstruction of a federal investigation
        18 U.S.C. Sec 1518 (2001), obstruction of a criminal health care investigation

Perjury:
        18 U.S.C. Sec 1623 (2001), perjury

[78] Mary Twomey, Mary Joy Quinn, and Emily Dakin, "From Behind Closed Doors: Shedding Light on Elder Abuse and Domestic Violence in Late Life," *Journal of the Center for Families, Children and the Courts* 6 (2005): 73–80.

[79] American Bar Association Commission on Law and Aging, *Information about Laws Related to Elder Abuse* (Washington, DC: National Center on Elder Abuse, 2005). Available at http://www.ncea.aoa.gov/ncearoot/Main_Site/pdf/publication/InformationAboutLawsRelatedtoElderAbuse.pdf.

[80] Ibid.

[81] See, for example, *United States v. Crawford, No. 4:1998cr00219* (E.D. Ark. Mar. 15, 2000); *United States v. Turner, no. 4:1998cr00215* (E.D. Ark. Mar. 15, 2000).

[82] Chisun Lee, A. C. Thompson, and Carl Byker, "Gone Without a Case: Suspicious Elder Deaths Rarely Investigated" (*FRONTLINE*, December 21, 2011). Available at http://www.pbs.org/wgbh/pages/frontline/criminal-justice/post-mortem/gone-without-a-case-suspicious-elder-deaths-rarely-investigated/.

[83] See Marie-Therese Connolly, "Federal Law Enforcement In Long Term Care," *Journal of Health Care Law and Policy*, 4, no. 2 (2002).

[84] American Prosecutors Research Institute, "Protecting America's Senior Citizens: What Local Prosecutors Are Doing to Fight Elder Abuse (Special Topic Series)," (Alexandria, VA: American Prosecutors Research Institute, 2003). Available at http://www.ndaa.org/pdf/protecting_ americas_senior_citizens_2003.pdf.

[85] Philip Bulman, "Elder Abuse Emerges From the Shadows of Public Consciousness" *NIJ Journal*, 265 (2010): 4–7. Available at https://www.ncjrs.gov/pdffiles1/nij/229883.pdf.

[86] Peter G. Lomhoff and Russell S. Balisok, *California Elder Law Litigation: An Advocate's Guide* (Oakland, CA: Continuing Education of The Bar, 2007).

[87] John F. Schnelle, Sandra F. Simmons, Charlene Harrington, Mary Cadogan, Emily Garcia, and Barbara Bates-Jensen. "Relationship of Nursing Home Staffing to Quality of Care," *Health Services Research*, 39, no. 2 (2004): 225–50.

[88] Minority Staff Special Investigations Division, *Abuse of Residents Is a Major Problem In U.S. Nursing Homes* (Washington, DC: US House of Representatives, 2001).

[89] Peggy Fox, reporting for 9 News Now (WUSA). Available at http://www.wusa9.com/news/local/story.aspx?storyid=113473.

[90] Daniel R. Levinson, *Nursing Facilities' Employment of Individuals with Criminal Convictions* (Washington, DC: Department of Health and Human Services, 2011). Available at http://oig.hhs.gov/oei/reports/oei-07-09-00110.pdf.

[91] David K Baugh, "Experiences of a Medicaid Nursing Home Entry Cohort," *Health Care Financing Review*, June 22, 1989. This study posits that the relative proportions and demographic characteristics of these two groups, the pattern of transfers between the inpatient hospital and the nursing home, and interstate variation in these dynamic factors are key determinants of nursing home utilization.

[92] The Online Survey Certification and Reporting (OSCAR) file was an administrative database of the Centers for Medicare and Medicaid Services for many years. Effective July 2012, survey data have been replaced with the Certification and Survey Provider Enhanced Reporting (CASPER) system and the Quality Improvement Evaluation System (QIES).

[93] Laurence Z. Rubenstein, "Preventing Falls in the Nursing Home," *Journal of the American Medical Association* 278, no. 7 (1997): 595–96.

[94] Laurence Z. Rubenstein, A.S. Robbins, B.L. Schulman, J. Rosado, D. Osterweil, and K.R. Josephson, "Falls and Instability in the Elderly, *Journal of the American Geriatrics Society* 36 (1988): 266–78.

[95] See, for example, F.K. Ejas, J.A. Jones, M.S. Rose, "Falls Among Nursing Home Residents: An Examination of Incident Reports Before and After Restraint Reduction Programs," *Journal of the American Geriatrics Society* 42, no. 9 (1994): 960–64. See also, L.Z. Rubenstein, K.R. Josephson, and A.S. Robbins, "Falls in the Nursing Home," *Annals of Internal Medicine*, 121 (1994): 442–51.

[96] Wayne A. Ray, Jo A. Taylor, Keith G. Meador, Purushottam B. Thapa, Anne K. Brown, Henry K. Kajihara, et al., "A Randomized Trial of a Consultation Service to Reduce Falls in Nursing Homes. *Journal of the American Medical Association* 278, no. 7 (1997): 557–62.

[97] See Cameron A. Mustard and Theresa Mayer, "Case-control Study of Exposure to Medication and the Risk of Injurious Falls Requiring Hospitalization Among Nursing Home Residents," *American Journal of Epidemiology* 145 (1997): 738–45 and W.A. Ray, P.B. Thapa, and P. Gideon, "Benzodiazepines and the Risk of Falls in Nursing Home Residents," *Journal of the American Geriatrics Society* 48, no. 6 (2000): 682–85.

[98] Gary S. Sorock, Patricia A. Quigley, Michelle K. Rutledge, et al., "Central Nervous System Medication Changes and Falls in Nursing Home Residents," *Geriatric Nursing* 30 (2009): 334–340.

[99] See Wayne A. Ray, Jo A. Taylor, Keith G. Meador, Purushottam B. Thapa, Anne K. Brown, Henry K. Kajihara, et al., "A Randomized Trial of a Consultation Service to Reduce Falls in Nursing Homes. *Journal of the American Medical Association* 278, no. 7 (1997): 557–62 and Mary Elizabeth Tinetti, "Factors Associated With Serious Injury During Falls By Ambulatory Nursing Home Residents," *Journal of the American Geriatrics Society* 35 (1987): 644–48.

[100] Sarah Greene Burger, Jeanie Kayser-Jones, and Julie Prince Bell, *Malnutrition And Dehydration In Nursing Homes: Key Issues In Prevention And Treatment* (Washington, DC: National Citizens' Coalition for Nursing Home Reform, 2000).

[101] E. F. Furman, "Undernutrition in Older Adults Across the Continuum of Care," *Journal of Gerontological Nursing* 32, no. 1 (2006): 22–27.

[102] S. D. Horn, S. A. Bender, N. Bergstrom, et al., "Description of the National Pressure Ulcer Long-Term Care Study," *Journal of the American Geriatric Society* 50, no. 11 (2002): 1816–25

[103] Nicholas G. Castle and John Engberg, "The Influence Of Staffing Characteristics On Quality Of Care in Nursing Homes," *Health Services Research* 42, no. 5 (2007): 1822–47.

Eric Collier and Charlene Harrington, "Staffing Characteristics, Turnover Rates, and Quality of Resident Care in Nursing Facilities," *Research in Gerontological Nursing* 1, no. 3 (2009): 157–170.

John F. Schnelle, Sandra F. Simmons, Charlene Harrington, Mary Cadogan, Emily Garcia, and Barbara M. Bates-Jensen, "Relationship of Nursing Home Staffing to Quality of Care?," *Health Services Research* 39, no. 2 (2004): 225–250.

[104] Abt Associates, *Appropriateness of Minimum Nurse Staffing Ratios in Nursing Homes: Report to Congress (Phase II Final)* (Baltimore, MD: US Centers for Medicare and Medicaid Services, 2001).

[105] Institute of Medicine (IOM), Committee on the Adequacy of Nurse Staffing in Hospitals and Nursing Homes, *Nursing Staff in Hospitals and Nursing Homes: Is it Adequate?* (Washington, DC: National Academy Press, 1996).

[106] Ning Jackie Zhang, Lynn Unruh, Rong Liu, and Thomas Wan, "Minimum Nurse Staffing Ratios for Nursing Homes," *Nursing Economics* 24, no. 2 (2006): 78–85, 93

[107] Charlotte Harrington and M. Millman, *Nursing Home Staffing Standards in State Statutes and Regulations* (San Francisco, CA: Henry J. Kaiser Family Foundation, 2001).

[108] Charlene Harrington et al., "Does Investor Ownership of Nursing Homes Compromise the Quality of Care?," *American Journal of Public Health* 91, no. 9 (2001): 1452–1455.

[109] Charlene Harrington, Helen Carrillo, Brandee Woleslagle Blank, and Teena O'Brian, *Nursing Facilities, Staffing, Residents and Facility Deficiencies, 2001-2007* (San Francisco: University of California, 2010).

[110] Charlene Harrington, Brian Olney, Helen Carrillo, and Taewoon Kang, "Nurse Staffing and Deficiencies in the Largest For-Profit Nursing Home Chains and Chains Owned by Private Equity Companies," *Health Services Research* 47, no. 1 (2012): 106–128.

[111] http://swz.salary.com/salarywizard/layouthtmls/swzl_compresult_national_HC07000412.html.

[112] Genesis HealthCare Proxy Statement. Available at http://www.sec.gov/Archives/edgar/data/1236736/000110465907017133/a07-

4061_1defm14a.htm.

[113] Medicare Payment Advisory Commission, *Medicare Payment Policy: Report to the Congress* (Washington, DC:, MedPac, 2009), 157–158. Available at http://medpac.gov/documents/Mar11_EntireReport.pdf.

[114] Medicare Payment Advisory Commission, *Medicare Payment Policy: Report to the Congress* (Washington, DC:, MedPac, 2009), 160–161. Available at http://www.medpac.gov/chapters/Mar09_Ch02D.pdf

[115] Ibid., 158.

[116] Walter Hamilton, "HCP to pay $6.1 billion for HCR ManorCare's Nursing Home Properties," *Los Angeles Times*, December 15, 2010.

[117] John Yedinak, "Wall Street Goes Long On Grannies," *The Economist*, March 25, 2010. Available at http://www.economist.com/node/17581666.

[118] Charles Duhigg, "At Many Homes, More Profit and Less Nursing," *New York Times*, September 23, 2007. Available at http://www.nytimes.com/2007/09/23/business/23nursing.html?pagewanted=all.

[119] General Accounting Office, *Providers Have Responded to Medicare Payment System by Changing Practices*, GAO-02-841 (Washington, DC: GAO, August 2002). Available at http://www.gao.gov/new.items/d02841.pdf.

[120] General Accounting Office, *Skilled Nursing Facilities: Available Data Show Average Nursing Staff Time Changed Little after Medicare Payment Increase*, GAO-03-176 (Washington, DC: GAO, November 2002), 3. Available at http://www.gao.gov/new.items/d03176.pdf.

[121] 76 Fed. Reg. 26364, at 36370 (May 6, 2011).

[122] Stuart Wright, "Early Alert Memorandum Report: Changes in Skilled Nursing Facilities Billing in Fiscal Year 2011" (OEI-02-09-0024) Early Alert Memorandum Report to Donald M. Berwick, Centers for Medicare and Medicaid Services, July 8, 2011. Available at http://oig.hhs.gov/oei/reports/oei-02-09-00204.pdf. The Government Accountability Office also recently documented high profit margins for skilled nursing facilities acquired by private investment firms. See: Government Accountability Office, *Nursing Homes: Private Investment Homes Sometimes Differed from Others in Deficiencies, Staffing, and Financial Performance*, GAO-11-571 (Washington, DC: GAO, July 2011), 34. Available at http://www.gao.gov/products/GAO-11-571.

[123] Christina Jewett and Agustin Armendariz, Nursing Homes Received Millions While Cutting Staff, Wages," *California Watch*, April 17, 2010. Available at http://californiawatch.org/health-and-welfare/nursing-homes-received-millions-while-cutting-staff-wages.

[124] Avalere Health LLC, "Skilled Nursing Facility Response to FY 2012 Medicare Payment Reductions: Survey Results." Available at http://www.aqnhc.org/images/2011-survey-results.pdf.

[125] Phil Moeller, "Nursing Homes Squeezed by Medicare Cuts," *US News*, August 8, 2011. Available at http://money.usnews.com/money/blogs/the-best-life/2011/08/08/nursing-homes-squeezed-by-medicare-cuts.

[126] Katharine Hsiao and Gerald McIntyre, "What You Need to Know About Advocacy for Limited-English-Proficient Elders," *Journal of Poverty Law and Policy, Clearinghouse Review* 42, no. 5–6 (2008): 301.

[127] Jennifer M. Ortman and Hyon B. Shin, "Language Projections: 2010 to 2020." Paper presented at the annual meeting of the American Sociological Association, Las Vegas, NV, 2011. Available at http://www.census.gov/hhes/socdemo/language/data/acs/Ortman_Shin_ASA2011_paper.pdf.

[128] Jane Perkins and Mara Youdelman, *Summary of State Law Requirements Addressing Language Needs in Health Care* (Washington, DC: National Health Law Program, 2008). Available at http://www.lawhelp.org/documents/383231nhelp.lep.state.law.chart.final.pdf.

[129] Ibid.

[130] Ibid.

[131] Chris Gastmans and Koen Milisen, "Use of Physical Restraint in Nursing Homes: Clinical- Ethical Considerations," *Journal of Medical* Ethics 32, no. 3 (2006): 148–152.

[132] Julie Applebye and Jack Gillum, "Fewer Care Facilities Use Restraints for Elderly Residents," *USA Today*, February 16, 2009. Available at http://www.usatoday.com/news/health/2009-02-16-nursing-home-restraints_N.htm.

[133] Agency for Healthcare Research and Quality, *National Healthcare Disparities Report, 2009*, (Washington, DC: Department of Health and Human Services, March 2010).

[134] Food and Drug Administration, "Public Health Advisory: Deaths with Antipsychotics in Elderly Patients with Behavioral Disturbances," April 11, 2005.

[135] Clive Ballard et al., "The Dementia Antipsychotic Withdrawal Trial (DART-AD): Long-Term Follow-up of a Randomised Placebo-Controlled Trial," *Lancet Neurology* 8, no. 2 (2009): 151–157, doi:10.1016/S1474-4422(08)70295-3.

[136] Food and Drug Administration, "Information for Healthcare Professionals: Conventional Antipsychotics," June 16, 2008.

[137] Centers for Medicare and Medicaid Services, "MDS Quality Measure/Indicator Report: Psychotropic Drug Use," July/September 2010, Measure 10_1_HI.

[138] Ibid., Measure 10_1_LO.

[139] Daniel R. Levinson, Inspector General, *Nursing Facility Assessments and Care Plans for Residents Receiving Atypical Antipsychotic Drugs* (Washington, DC:

Department of Health and Human Services, July 2012). Available at
http://oig.hhs.gov/oei/reports/oei-07-08-00151.pdf.

[140] GAO, *Nursing Homes: Federal Monitoring Surveys Demonstrate Continued Understatement of Serious Care Problems and CMS Oversight Weaknesses*, GAO-08-517 (Washington, DC: May 9, 2008).

[141] Ada-Helen Bayer and Leon Harper, *Fixing to Stay: A National Survey on Housing and Home Modification Issues* (Washington, DC: AARP, May 2000).

[142] Mathew Greenwald and Associates, *These Four Walls: Americans 45+ Talk About Home and Community* (Washington, DC: AARP, May 2003).

[143] John Hill, Caregiver Roulette: California Fails to Screen Those Who Care for the Elderly at Home (Sacramento, CA: California Senate Office Oversight and Outcomes, 2011). Available at
http://www3.senate.ca.gov/deployedfiles/vcm2007/senoversight/docs/2385.caregiver%20roulette.pdf.

[144] 42 U.S.C. § 3604(f)(3)(A).

[145] Centers for Disease Control and Prevention, National Center for Injury Prevention and Control, *Web-based Injury Statistics Query and Reporting System (WISQARS)*, Accessed November 30, 2010.

[146] Center for the Advanced Study of Aging Services, *UC Berkeley Villages Project: Evaluating an Innovative Approach for Aging in Place* (Berkeley, CA: UC Berkeley School of Social Welfare, 2011). Available at
http://cssr.berkeley.edu/research_units/casas/documents/CASAS_fall_2011.pdf.

[147] Louise A. Meret-Hanke, "Effects of the Program of All-Inclusive Care for the Elderly on Hospital Use," *The Gerontologist*, July 2011. doi: 10.1093/geront/gnr040

[148] Andrew F. Coburn and Elise J. Bolda, "Rural Elders and Long Term Care," *Western Journal of Medicine* 174, no. 3 (2001): 209–213.

[149] Karl Polzer, *Assisted Living State Regulatory Review* (Washington, DC: National Center for Assisted Living, 2011).

[150] Keren Brown Wilson, "Historical Evolution of Assisted Living in the United States, 1979 to the Present," *The Gerontologist* 47, no. 3 (2007), 8–22.

[151] Ibid.

[152] Rosalie A. Kane and Keren Brown Wilson, *Assisted Living In The United States: A New Paradigm For Residential Care For Frail Older Persons?* (Washington, DC: AARP, 1993).

[153] Keren Brown Wilson, "Historical Evolution of Assisted Living in the United States, 1979 to the Present," *The Gerontologist* 47, no. 3 (2007), 8–22.

[154] Robert Mollica, *State Assisted Living Policy: 2002* (Portland, ME: National Academy for State Health Policy, November 2002).

[155] See, for example: Florida Agency for Health Care Administration, *Nursing Home and Assisted Living Facility: Adverse Incidents & Notices of Intent Filed (Status Report)*, June 2003; Texas Department of Human Services, *Fiscal Year 2003: Long Term Care Regulatory Annual Report*, November 2003; Sue Seely, "Assisted Living: Federal and State Options for Affordability, Quality of Care, and Consumer Protection," *Bifocal* 23, no. 1 (2001): 1.

[156] Kevin McCoy and Julie Appleby, "Problems with Staffing, Training Can Cost Lives, *USA Today*, May 28, 2004. Available at http://www.usatoday.com/money/industries/health/2004-05-26-assisted-day2_x.htm.

[157] Catherine Hawes, "Elder Abuse in Residential Long-Term Care Facilities: What is Known and What Information is Needed?, unpublished manuscript cited in Marie-Therese Connolly, "Federal Law Enforcement In Long Term Care," *Journal of Health Care Law and Policy*, 4, no. 2 (2002).

[158] Ibid.

[159] Administration on Aging, *National Ombudsman Reporting System Data FY 2002* (Washington, DC: Department of Health and Human Services).

[160] General Accounting Office, *Assisted Living: Examples of State Efforts to Improve Consumer Protections*, GAO-04-684 (Washington, DC: GAO, April 2004).

[161] See: General Accounting Office, *Assisted Living: Quality-of-Care and Consumer Protection Issues in Four States*, GAO/HEHS-99-27 (Washington, DC: GAO, April 26, 1999) and General Accounting Office, *Consumer Protection and Quality-of-Care Issues in Assisted Living*, GAO/HEHS-97-93 (Washington, DC: GAO, May 15, 1997).

[162] See, for example, National Academy of Elder Law Attorneys, *White Paper on Assisted Living* (Tucson, AZ, 2001) and Deanna Okrent and Virginia Dize, *Ombudsman Advocacy Challenges in Assisted Living: Outreach and Discharge* (Washington, DC: National Association of State Units on Aging, March 2001).

[163] See section 1.5 of National Academy for State Health Policy, *State Assisted Living Policy: 2002* (Portland, ME, November 2002).

[164] Ziegler Capital Markets, *Ziegler National CCRC Listing and Profile* (Chicago, IL: Ziegler, 2009).

[165] Jane E. Zarem, ed., *Today's Continuing Care Retirement Community* (CCRC Task Force, July 2010). Available at https://www.seniorshousing.org/filephotos/research/CCRC_whitepaper.pdf.

[166] Government Accountability Office, *Continuing Care Retirement Communities Can Provide Benefits, but Not Without Some Risk*, GAO-10-611 (Washington, DC: GAO, July 21, 2010).

[167] Mike Cherney, "'Senior' Debt's New Appeal: Investors Warm To Bonds Tied to Retirement Homes," *Wall Street Journal*, February 8, 2012. Available at http://online.wsj.com/article/SB10001424052970203833004577249570046437

482.html.

[168] Ibid.

[169] Kelly Greene, "Continuing-Care Retirement Communities: Weighing the Risks," *Wall Street Journal*, August 7, 2010. Available at http://online.wsj.com/article/SB10001424052748704499604575407290112356 422.html#articleTabs%3Darticle.

[170] Malaz Boustani, Sheryl Zimmerman, Christianna S. Williams, Ann L. Gruber-Baldini, Lea Watson, Peter S. Reed, and Philip D. Sloane, "Characteristics Associated with Behavioral Symptoms Related to Dementia in Long-Term Care Residents," *Gerontologist* 45, no. 1 (2005): 56–61. Available at http://www.alz.org/national/documents/grnt_056_061.pdf.

[171] A. Rosenblatt, Q. Samus, C. Steele, A. Baker, M. G. Harper, J. Brandt, et al., "The Maryland Assisted Living Study: Prevalence, Recognition, and Treatment of Dementia and Other Psychiatric Disorders in the Assisted Living Population of Central Maryland," *Journal of the American Geriatrics Society* 52, no. 10 (2004): 1618–1625.

[172] Ann L. Gruber-Baldini, Sheryl Zimmerman, Malaz Boustani, Lea C. Watson, Christianna S. Williams, Peter S. Reed, "Characteristics Associated with Depression in Long-Term Care Residents with Dementia," *Gerontologist* 45, special issue no. 1 (2005): 50–55.

[173] Malaz Boustani, Sheryl Zimmerman, Christianna S. Williams, Ann L. Gruber-Baldini, Lea Watson, Peter S. Reed, and Philip D. Sloane, "Characteristics Associated with Behavioral Symptoms Related to Dementia in Long-Term Care Residents," *Gerontologist* 45, no. 1 (2005): 56–61.

[174] Marianne Smith, Kathleen C. Buckwalter, Hyunwook Kang, Vicki Ellingrod, and Susan K. Schultz, "Dementia Care In Assisted Living: Needs And Challenges," *Issues in Mental Health Nursing* 29, no. 8 (2008): 817–838. Available at http://www.ncbi.nlm.nih.gov/pmc/articles/PMC3093103/.

[175] Assisted Living Workgroup, *Assuring Quality in Assisted Living: Guidelines for Federal and State Policy, State Regulation, and Operations*" (A Report to the US Senate Special Committee on Aging), April 2003.

[176] The foundation of Person-Centered Care is the work of Professor Tom Kitwood, who headed the Bradford Dementia Group in the United Kingdom from 1992 to 1998.

[177] Jane Tilly and Peter Reed, eds., *Dementia Care Practice Recommendations for Assisted Living Residences and Nursing Homes* (Chicago, IL: Alzheimer's Association, 2009).

[178] Ibid.

[179] Gilberte Van Rensbergen and Tim Nawrot, "Medical Conditions of Nursing Home Admissions," *BMC Geriatrics* 10 (2010): 46. doi:10.1186/1471-2318-10-46

[180] Cynthia L. Leibson, Jeanine E. Ransom, Robert D. Brown, Michael O'Fallon, Steven Hass, Jack P. Whisnant, "Stroke-Attributable Nursing Home Use: A Population-Based Study," *Neurology* 51, no. 1 (1998): 163–168.

[181] Edward C. Jauch, "Acute Stroke Management," *eMedicine.com* (2002): 1–32. Available at http://www.emedicine.com/neuro/topic9.htm.

[182] J. David Curb, Richard D. Abbot, C. J. Maclean, Beatriz L. Rodriquez, C. M. Burchfiel, D. S. Sharp, G. Webster Ross, K. Yano, "Age Related Changes in Stroke Risk in Men with Hypertension and Normal Blood Pressure," *Stroke* 27, no. 5 (1996): 819–24.

[183] J. P. Mohr, Gregory W. Albers, Pierre Amarenco, Viken L. Babikian, Jose Biller, Robin L. Brey, et al., "American Heart Association Prevention Conference IV: Prevention and Rehabilitation of Stroke," *Stroke* 28, no. 7 (1997): 1501–1506.

[184] Todd J. Anderson, "Assessment and Treatment of Endothelial Dysfunction in Humans," *Journal of the American College of Cardiology* 34, no. 3 (1993): 631–38.

[185] Frank D. Kolodgie, Allen P. Burke, Gaku Nakazawa, and Renu Virmani, "Thickening: The Key to Understanding Early Plaque Progression in Human Atherosclerotic Disease?" *Arteriosclerosis, Thrombosis & Vascular Biology* 27, no. 5 (2007): 986–989.

[186] Stephen N. Macciocchi, Paul T. Diamond, Wayne M. Alves, and Tracie Mertz, "Ischemic Stroke: Relation of Age, Lesion Location, and Initial Neurologic Deficit to Functional Outcome," *Archives of Physical and Medical Rehabilitation* 79, no. 10 (1998): 1255–1257.

[187] Wayne Rosamond et al., "Heart Disease and Stroke Statistics, 2008 Update: A Report From the American Heart Association Statistics Committee and Stroke Statistics Subcommittee," *Circulation* 117, no. 4 (2007): e25–e146.

[188] Christopher B. Brady, Avron Spiro, III, and J. Michael Gaziano, "Effects of Age and Hypertension Status on Cognition: The Veterans Affairs Normative Aging Study," *Neuropsychology* 19, no. 6 (2005): 770–777.

[189] John Hopkins, *Hypertension (High Blood Pressure) and Stroke*. Available at http://www.johnshopkinshealthalerts.com/alerts_index/hypertension_stroke/21-1.html.

[190] Frank D. Kolodgie, Herman K. Gold, Allen P. Burke, et al., "Intraplaque Hemorrhage and Progression of Coronary Atheroma," *New England Journal of Medicine* 349, no. 24 (2003): 2316–25.

[191] Peter M. Nilsson, "Reducing the Risk of Stroke in Elderly Patients with Hypertension: A Critical Review of the Efficacy of Antihypertensive Drug," *Drugs & Aging* 22, no. 6 (2005): 517–24.

[192] American Heart Association, *Physical Activity and Blood Pressure*. Available at http://www.heart.org/HEARTORG/Conditions/HighBloodPressure/PreventionTreatmentofHighBloodPressure/Physical-Activity-and-Blood-Pressure_UCM_301882_Article.jsp.

[193] Barbro B. Johansson, "Hypertension Mechanisms Causing Stroke," *Clinical and Experimental Pharmacology and Physiology* 26, no. 7 (1999): 563–56.

[194] Cleveland Clinic, *Disease Management Project Medicine Index* (Online Medical Reference Guide). Available at http://www.clevelandclinicmeded.com/medicalpubs/diseasemanagement/.

[195] See, for example, Thomas Almdal, Henrik Scharling, Jan Skov Jensen, and Henrik Vestergaard, "The Independent Effect of Type 2 Diabetes Mellitus on Ischemic Heart Disease, Stroke, and Death," *Archives of Internal Medicine* 164, no. 13 (2004): 1422–1426; Henrik S. Jorgensen, Hirofumi Nakayama, Hans O. Raaschou, and Tom S. Olsen, "The Copenhagen Stroke Study: Stroke in Patients with Diabetes," *Stroke* 25, no. 10 (1994): 1977–1984; Susan P. Laing, Anthony J. Swerdlow, Lucy M. Carpenter, et al., "Mortality From Cerebrovascular Disease in a Cohort Of 23,000 Patients With Insulin-Treated Diabetes," *Stroke* 34, no. 2 (2003): 418–421.

[196] Diabetes Association, *Diabetes: Heart Disease and Stroke*. Available at http://www.diabetes.org/diabetes-heart-disease-stroke.jsp.

[197] Bantwal Suresh Baliga and Jesse Weinberger, "Diabetes and Stroke: Part One— Risk Factors and Pathophysiology," *Current Cardiology Reports* 8, no. 1 (2006): 23–8.

[198] Henrik S. Jorgensen, Hirofumi Nakayama, Hans O. Raaschou, and Tom S. Olsen, "The Copenhagen Stroke Study: Stroke in Patients with Diabetes," *Stroke* 25, no. 10 (1994): 1977–1984.

[199] Ralph L. Sacco, Philip A. Wolf, and Philip B. Gorelick, "Risk Factors and Their Management for Stroke Prevention: Outlook for 1999 and Beyond," *Neurology* 53, no. 7, sup. 4 (1999): S15–24.

[200] Clara Sanz, Jean-Francois Gautier, and Helene Hanaire, "Physical Exercise for the Prevention and Treatment of Type 2 Diabetes," *Diabetes and Metabolism* 36, no. 5 (2010): 346–51.

[201] Timothy S. Church, Steven N. Blair, Shannon Cocreham, et al., "Effects of Aerobic and Resistance Training on Hemoglobin A_{1c} Levels in Patients With Type 2 Diabetes," *JAMA*, 304, no. 20 (2010): 2253–62. doi: 10.1001/jama.2010.1710

[202] Ronald J. Sigal, Glen P. Kenny, David H. Wasserman, Carmen Castaneda-Sceppa, and Russell D. White, "Physical Activity/Exercise and Type 2 Diabetes: A Consensus Statement From The American Diabetes Association," *Diabetes Care* 29, no. 6 (2006): 1433–38.

[203] Gang Hu, Cinzia Sarti, Pekka Jousilahti, Markku Peltonen, Qing Qiao, Riitta Antikainen, and Jaakko Tuomilehto, "The Impact of History of Hypertension and Type 2 Diabetes at Baseline on the Incidence of Stroke and Stroke Mortality," *Stroke* 36, no. 12 (2005): 2538–43.

[204] See, for example: Scott M. Grundy, James I. Cleeman, C. Noel Bairey Merz, et al., "Implications of Recent Clinical Trials for the National Cholesterol Education

Program Adult Treatment Panel III Guidelines," *Circulation* 110, no. 2 (2004): 227–239; Alice H. Lichtenstein, Lawrence J. Appel, Michael Brands, et al., "Diet and Lifestyle Recommendations Revision 2006: A Scientific Statement From the American Heart Association Nutrition Committee," *Circulation* 114 (2006): 82–96; J. P. Mohr, Dennis W. Choi, James C. Grotta, Bryce Weir, and Phillip A. Wolfe, *Stroke: Pathophysiology, Diagnosis, and Management* (New York: Churchill Livingstone, 4th ed., 2004).

[205] National Heart, Lung, and Blood Institute, *Your Guide to Lowering High Blood Pressure*. Available at www.nhlbi.nih.gov/hbp.

[206] Although high cholesterol contributes to atherosclerosis and the risk of ischemic stroke, elevated serum cholesterol (your total cholesterol level) has been considered a poor predictor of stroke and is associated negatively with hemorrhagic stroke risk. (See Benjamin J. Ansell, "Cholesterol, Stroke Risk, and Stroke Prevention," *Current Atherosclerosis Reports* 2, no. 2 (2000): 92–96.) Indeed, the results of a recent British study suggest that the connection between cholesterol levels and stroke may be attenuated. The analysis of 61 studies, which consisted of a data survey on almost 900,000 adults who had no heart disease at the start of the studies, found that for people in their seventies and eighties, high cholesterol actually lowered stroke risk, even as it boosted the odds for heart attack. (See Prospective Studies Collaboration et al., "Blood Cholesterol and Vascular Mortality by Age, Sex, and Blood Pressure: A Meta-Analysis of Individual Data from 61 Prospective Studies with 55,000 Vascular Deaths," *Lancet* 370, no. 9602 (2007): 1829–39.)

[207] Etienne Joosten et al., "Metabolic Evidence That Deficiencies of Vitamin B-12 (Cobalamin), Folate, and Vitamin B-6 Occur Commonly in Elderly People," *American Journal of Clinical Nutrition* 58, no. 3 (1993): 468–76.

[208] Hyun W. Baik and Robert M. Russell, "Vitamin B_{12} Deficiency In The Elderly," *Annual Review of Nutrition* 19 (1999): 357–377. doi:10.1146/annurev.nutr.19.1.357

[209] Victor Herbert, "Vitamin B-12: Plant Sources, Requirements, and Assay," *American Journal of Clinical Nutrition* 48, no. 3 supp (1988): 852–58.

[210] B. Shane, "Folic Acid, Vitamin B-12, and Vitamin B-6," in *Biochemical and Physiological Aspects of Human Nutrition*, ed. Martha H. Stipanuk (Philadelphia: W.B. Saunders Co., 2000), 483–518.

[211] Hyun W. Baik and Robert M. Russell, "Vitamin B_{12} Deficiency In The Elderly," *Annual Review of Nutrition* 19 (1999): 357–377. doi:10.1146/annurev.nutr.19.1.357

[212] Petra Verhoef, Frans J. Kok, Dick A. Kruyssen, et al., "Plasma Total Homocysteine, B Vitamins, and Risk of Coronary Atherosclerosis," *Arteriosclerosis, Thrombosis, and Vascular Biology* 17, no. 5 (1997): 989–95.

[213] See, for example: Jeremy D. Kark, Jacob Selhub, Bella Adler, et al., "Nonfasting Plasma Total Homocysteine Level and Mortality in Middle-Aged and Elderly Men

and Women in Jerusalem," *Annals of Internal Medicine* 131, no. 5 (1999), 321–330; Jacob Selhub, Paul F. Jacques, Irwin H. Rosenberg, et al., "Serum Total Homocysteine Concentrations in the Third National Health and Nutrition Examination Survey (1991–1994)," *Annals of Internal Medicine* 131, no. 5 (1999): 331–339; Andrew G. Bostom, Irwin H. Rosenberg, Halit Silbershatz, et al., "Non-Fasting Plasma Total Homocysteine Levels and Stroke Incidence in Elderly Persons: The Framingham Study," *Annals of Internal Medicine* 131, no. 5 (1999): 352–355; John W. Eikelboom, Eva Lonn, Jacques Genest, Jr., et al., "Homocyst(e)ine and Cardiovascular Disease: A Critical Review of the Epidemiologic Evidence, *Annals of Internal Medicine* 131, no. 5 (1999): 363–375.

[214] Jacques Genest, Jr., Marie-Chantal Audelin, and Eva Lonn, "Homocysteine: To Screen and Treat or To Wait and See?," *Canadian Medical Association Journal* 163, no. 1 (2000): 37–38.

[215] National Institute of Health, *Alzheimer's Disease Fact Sheet*. Available at http://www.nia.nih.gov/alzheimers/publication/alzheimers-disease-fact-sheet

[216] Elizabeth P. Helzner, José A. Luchsinger, Nikolaos Scarmeas, et al., "Contribution of Vascular Risk Factors to the Progression in Alzheimer Disease," *Archives of Neurology* 66, no. 3 (2009) 343–48.

[217] Fred H. Gage, "Neurogenesis in the Adult Brain," *Journal of Neuroscience* 22, no. 3 (2002): 612–613; Robert P. Friedland, Thomas Fritsch, Kathleen A. Smyth, et al., "Patients With Alzheimer's Disease Have Reduced Activities in Midlife Compared With Healthy Control-Group Members," *Proceedings of the National Academy of Sciences of the USA* 98, no. 6 (2001): 3440–45; Stanley J. Colcombe, Kirk I. Erickson, Naftali Raz, et al., "Aerobic Fitness Reduces Brain Tissue Loss in Aging Humans," *Journal of Gerontology* 58A, no. 2 (2003): 176–180; Wendy A. Rogers and Arthur D. Fisk, eds., *Human Factors Interventions for the Health Care of Older Adults* (Mahwah, NJ: Lawrence Erlbaum, 2001).

[218] Kim N. Green, Lauren M. Billings, Benno Roozendaal, James L. McGaugh, and Frank M. LaFerla, "Glucocorticoids Increase Amyloid- and Tau Pathology in a Mouse Model of Alzheimer's Disease," *The Journal of Neuroscience* 26, no. 35 (2006): 9047–56.

[219] Ibid.

[220] Ibid.

[221] Rush University Medical Center, *Foods that May Help Prevent Alzheimer's Disease.* Available at http://www.rush.edu/rumc/page-1102020578338.html. See also Yian Gu, Jeri W. Nieves, Yaakov Stern, Jose A. Luchsinger, and Nikolaos Scarmeas, "Food Combination and Alzheimer Disease Risk: A Protective Diet," *Archives of Neurology* 67, no. 6 (2010): 699–706.

[222] Jose A. Luchsinger, James M. Noble, and Nikolaos Scarmeas, "Diet and Alzheimer's Disease," *Current Neurology and Neuroscience Reports* 7, no. 5 (2007): 366–72. doi: 10.1007/s11910-007-0057-8

[223] Mary E. Tinetti and Christianna S. Williams, "Falls, Injuries Due to Falls, and

the Risk of Admission to a Nursing Home," *New England Journal of Medicine* 337, no. 18 (1997): 1279–84.

[224] George F. Fuller, "Falls in the Elderly," *American Family Physician* 61, no. 7 (2000): 2159–68.

[225] Lesley Gillespie, M. Clare Robertson, William J. Gillespie, Sarah E. Lamb, Simon Gates, Robert G. Cumming, and Brian H. Rowe, *Interventions For Preventing Falls in Older People Living in the Community (Review)* (Melbourne, Australia: The Cochrane Collaboration & Wiley, 2009). doi: 10.1002/14651858.CD007146.pub2.

[226] Kuei-Min Chen and Mariah Snyder, "A Research-Based Use of Tai Chi Therapy as a Nursing Intervention," *Journal of Holistic Nursing* 17, no. 3 (1999): 267–279

[227] Deborah P. Schoenfelder, "A Fall Prevention Program for Elderly Individuals: Exercise in Long Term Settings," *Journal of Gerontological Nursing* 26, no. 3 (2000): 43–51

[228] American Academy of Neurology, "Depression may Nearly Double Your Risk of Developing Dementia" (Press Release, July 6, 2010).

[229] Science Daily, "Depression Increases Risk of Alzheimer's Disease" (Press Release, April 10, 2008), available at http://www.sciencedaily.com/releases/2008/04/080407162400.htm; Science Daily, "Obesity and Depression May Be Linked" (Press Release, June 6, 2008), available at http://www.sciencedaily.com/releases/2008/06/080602152913.htm; Science Daily, "Depression Tied to Higher Risk of Heart Disease Death" (Press Release, January 5, 2005), available at http://www.sciencedaily.com/releases/2005/01/050105065411.htm.

[230] Greg J. Lamberty and Linas A. Bieliauskas, "Distinguishing Between Depression and Dementia in the Elderly: A Review of Neuropsychological Findings," *Archives of Clinical Neuropsychology* 8, no. 2 (1993): 149–170.

[231] Some of the these triggers have been previously identified in my e-book, *Seven Triggers of Mental Health Decline in Seniors and How to Combat Them Forever.*

[232] Bernice Bratter, Helen Dennis, and Lahni Baruck, *Project Renewment* (New York: Simon & Schuster, 2008).

[233] Pekka Martikainen and Tapani Valkonen, "Mortality After the Death of a Spouse: Rates and Causes of Death in a Large Finnish Cohort," *American Journal of Public Health* 86, no. 8, part 1 (1996): 1087–93.

[234] For example, for general information about sleep, see http://science.education.nih.gov/supplements/nih3/sleep/guide/info-sleep.htm; for information on sleep disorders, see http://health.nih.gov/topic/SleepDisorders; and for information about sleep and aging, see http://nihseniorhealth.gov/sleepandaging/aboutsleep/01.html.

[235] Elizabeth Alicandri, Mark Robinson, and Tim Penney, "Designing Highways with Older Drivers in Mind," *Public Roads* 62, no. 6 (1999). Available at http://www.tfhrc.gov/pubrds/mayjun99/olddrvrs.htm.

[236] David F. Preusser, Allan F. Williams, Susan A. Ferguson, Robert G. Ullmer, and Helen B. Weinstein, "Fatal Crash Risk for Older Drivers at Intersections," *Accident Analysis and Prevention* 30, no. 2 (1998): 151–59.

[237] Office of Program Development and Evaluation, Traffic Safety Programs, *Addressing the Safety Issues Related to Younger and Older Drivers: A Report to Congress* (Washington, DC: US Department of Transportation, 1993), 16. Available at http://www.nhtsa.gov/people/injury/olddrive/pub/yorept.html.

[238] Highway Loss Data Institute, *Older Drivers: Licensing Renewal Provisions* (Arlington, VA: Insurance Institute for Highway Safety, 2012). Available at http://www.iihs.org/laws/olderdrivers.aspx.

[239] MetLife Mature Market Institute, *The 2011 MetLife Market Survey of Nursing Home, Assisted Living, Adult Day Services, and Home Care Costs* (Westport, CT: Mature Market Institute, 2011). Available at http://www.metlife.com/mmi/research/2011-market-survey-long-term-care-costs.html#findings.

[240] MetLife Mature Market Institute, *Market Survey of Long-Term Care Costs* (Westport, CT: Mature Market Institute, 2009). Available at http://www.metlife.com/assets/cao/mmi/publications/studies/2010/mmi-2010-market-survey-long-term-care-costs.pdf#findings.

[241] Christine Dugas, "Bankruptcy Rising Among Seniors," *USA TODAY*, June 16, 2008. Available at http://www.usatoday.com/money/perfi/retirement/2008-06-16-bankruptcy-seniors_N.htm.

[242] John Pottow, "The Rise in Elder Bankruptcy Filings and the Failure of U.S. Bankruptcy Law," *Elder Law Journal* 19, no. 1 (2011): 119–57.

[243] Jeffrey A. Sonnenfeld, "Dealing with the Aging Workforce," *Harvard Business Review* 56, no. 6 (1978): 81.

[244] Jessica Collison, *SHRM/NOWCC/CED Older Workers Survey* (Alexandria, VA: Society for Human Resource Management, 2003).

[245] At the same time, we must be mindful of our children and grandchildren and the huge wealth gap between younger and older Americans. According to 2011 census data, older people today have 47 times more money than younger people, and they have 42 percent more wealth than their same-aged counterparts did in 1984, while the younger generation has 68 percent less than theirs. With the older generation staying in the workforce longer and then relying on social security (the continued funding of which is on the younger generation's back) we could be in store for a serious age war. Those in the younger generation—including my two older stepsons—face heavily impacted classes at their respective universities and have few job opportunities. If they cannot afford college, they might even forgo higher education because of the cost of student loans. Those who have graduated and have started families cannot afford housing. When engaging in public debate about senior services and resources, we must keep this growing gap in mind and strive to create equity across the generations. Beyond the moral implications, from

a practical standpoint it may help us avoid a clash that we may not be able to withstand.

[246] For more information, see the publication entitled, "How Work Affects Your Benefits" (SSA Publication No. 05-10069, ICN 467005, March 2012).

[247] For more information, visit the website of the American Association for Long-Term Care Insurance (http://www.aaltci.org).

[248] Government Accountability Office, *Life Insurance Settlements: Regulatory Inconsistencies May Pose a Number of Challenges*, GAO-10-775 (Washington, DC: GAO, July 2010). Available at http://www.gao.gov/new.items/d10775.pdf

[249] See Section 1917(b)(2) of the Social Security Act and Section 3810.A.5 of the State Medicaid Manual.

[250] Les Leopold, "A Single Hedge-Fund Hustler Makes More Than 85,000 Teachers: Why Are Our Priorities So Messed Up?," *AlterNet*, March 23, 2012. Available at http://www.alternet.org/story/154671/a_single_hedge-fund_hustler_makes_more_than_85%2C000_teachers%3A_why_are_our_priorities_so_messed_up/.

Index